Xtreme
Sports Training
Renegade Style
Coach Davies

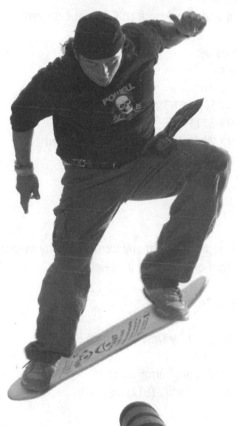

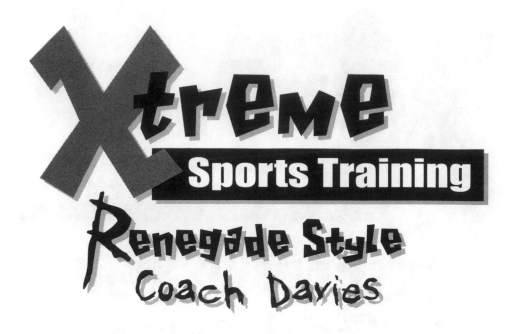

Xtreme Sports Training
Renegade Style
Coach Davies

Published in the United States by:
Dragon Door Publications, Inc
P.O. Box 4381, St. Paul, MN 55104
Tel: (651) 487-2180 • Fax: (651) 487-3954
Credit card orders: 1-800-899-5111
Email: dragondoor@aol.com • Website: www.dragondoor.com

ISBN: 0-938045-51-2

This edition first published in July 2003

Printed in the United States of America

Book design, Illustrations and cover by Derek Brigham
Website http//www.dbrigham.com
Tel/Fax: (612) 827-3431 • Email: dbrigham@visi.com
Photographs of the author by Don Pitlik: (612) 252-6797

DISCLAIMER

The author and publisher of this material are not responsible in any manner whatsoever for any injury that may occur through following the instructions contained in this material. The activities, physical and otherwise, described herein for informational purposes only, may be too strenuous or dangerous for some people and the reader(s) should consult a physician before engaging in them.

Table of Contents

Chapter 3
Xtreme Agility—How to Achieve
Cat-Like Balance and Super-Quick Reaction Times

The importance of improving agility for performance success...sport-specific skills...why the Renegade approach uses Swiss balls and balance boards.

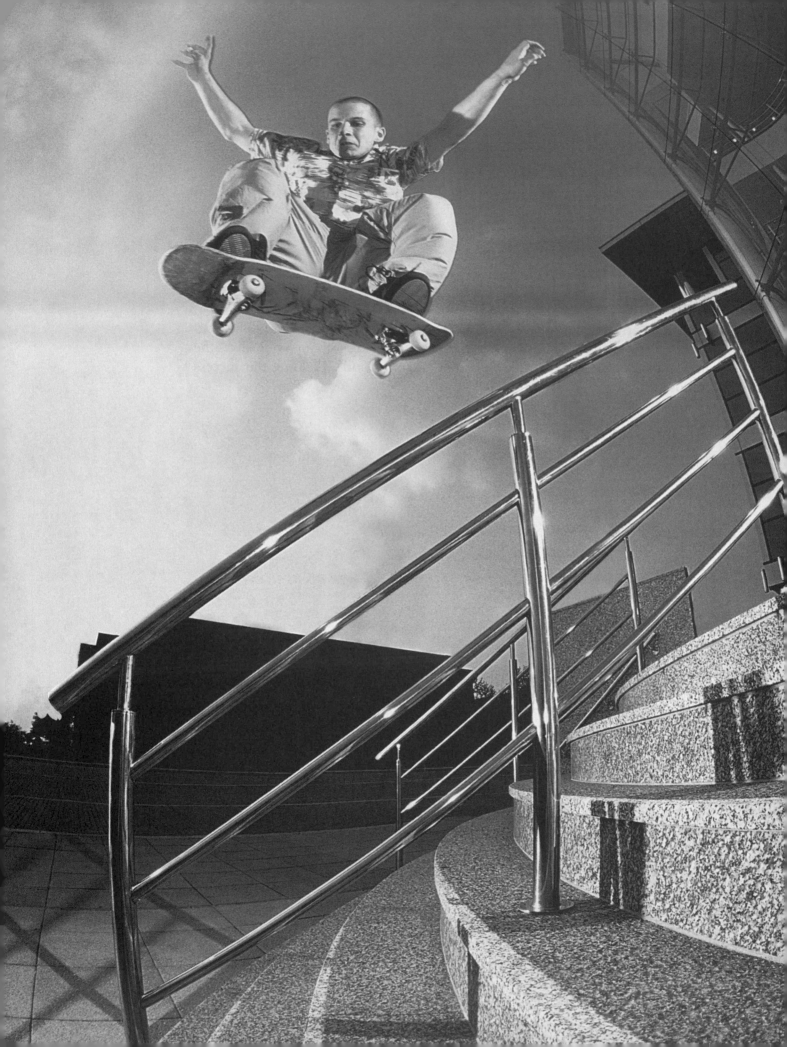

The Renegade Creed

A choice for those without choices,
where victory is the only option.

The mission is simple: to seize the opportunity, deny the
competition, and establish dominance.

The work of Renegades is for neither the soft
nor the weak. Renegades are relentless in
their attack with total vicious-like commitment
to their objectives.

Renegade Training breeds explosive, powerful, and
fast athletes who dictate the ebb and flow of competition such
that they are victorious.

If you are ready for the challenge—ready to master your
athletic destiny—then enter the world of Renegade Training.

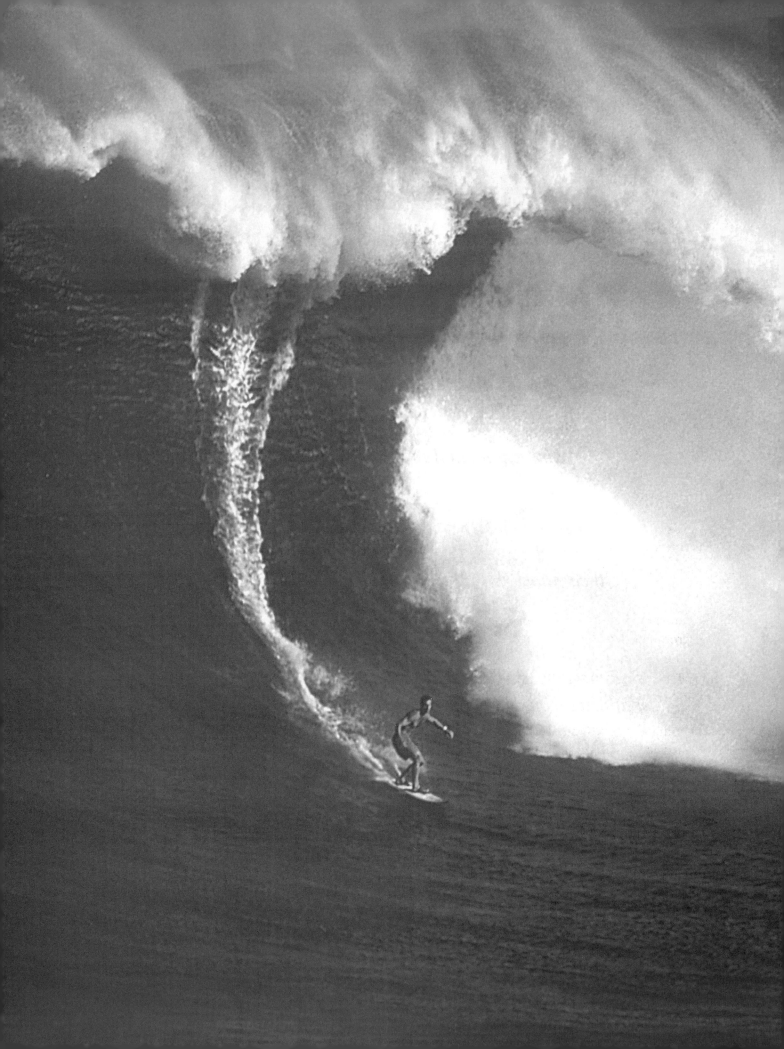

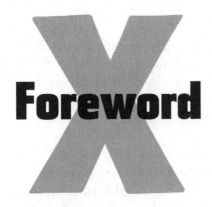

Foreword

By Hunter Joslin

Extreme Sports have been around for a long time and yet the general public's recognition only really began in 1995, with the first televised coverage of the ESPN X-Games, which ballyhooed the term "Extreme" and gave it worldwide acceptance. An extreme athlete—regardless of their particular choice amongst the many under the broad umbrella of Extreme Sports—is an individual who relentlessly pursues the natural high resulting from adrenaline producing sports. These adrenaline junkies have chosen a physical activity that is intensely self-rewarding, requiring a singular resolve to rely on ones ability to perform totally outside the realm of team sports. The risks are high and the reward is absolute self-satisfaction.

I started surfing and skateboarding in 1965 without any thought to being an extreme athlete, because growing up in South Florida my world was devoid of hills and big surf. This all changed when I started traveling and experiencing more radical conditions—experiencing the hills of Southern California, the Rocky Mountains, Hawaiian waves, and Indonesian barrels! It was during this same time that I was using the first prototypes of the Indo Board for my own training unbeknownst to the rest of the world. I designed the Original Indo Board in 1976 and it has since become regarded as the quintessential tool for surfing and other board sports training.

I entered the Extreme sports arena in 1977 managing a skatepark in West Palm Beach, Florida. This led to managing the legendary SIMS East Coast Skateboard Team 77-78, ending up in California cruising with Tom Inouye, Chris Strople and Brad Strandlund skating the parks from San Diego to Oxnard. I worked as MC for the 1st Hester Pro Bowl Series, playing an important part in the birth of vertical skateboard competition.

In 1979 I traveled to Hawaii living with Larry Bertlemann and Family for 2 months before heading off to Australia with the Town and Country Surf Team. It was during this trip that I was introduced to the International Professional

Surfing Tour, where I began my careful study of the common denominators that separated the best surfers in the World from us mere mortals. These theories are the basis of my Indo Board training for all board sports, whether it be Surf, Skate, Snow or Wake but also for the heavy demands on the Mountain Bike trails or BMX courses.

In 1984 I started announcing Professional Surfing events working in Australia, California, Puerto Rico, Costa Rica, Barbados, and all over the East Coast. The demand for my historical background and key analytical insight into the sport is such that to date I have announced over 125 professional events.

Surfing created skateboarding as a land-based simulation of the water born sport. As the equipment changed and evolved, the direction of these sports took a new, more radical course. Shorter surfboards and urethane wheels opened the door to the vertical direction that dominates these disciplines today. Skating progressed at an incredible pace, quickly leaving surfing behind on a performance level as well as on a popularity scale.

Skateable terrain of concrete and asphalt wasn't confined to the coast, which, combined with the reasonable cost of equipment, attracted participants from all neighborhoods regardless of age, race and income brackets. Skateparks and empty swimming pools unlocked the door to "extreme" skating with skateboarders starting to explore riding with only air under their wheels as they realized the combination of speed and vertical trajectory literally allowed them to fly through the air.

Surfers in the meantime were left to wonder how they could find the same lines out in the waves. Around the same time, the two-wheeled world heard the call and simple bike riding evolved into the artistry of the flatlander and the thriving pulse of BMX, MTB or Moto. The sporting world has never looked back and will never be the same.

The reality that surfing is the integration of the surfer, the board and the ever-changing wave, while skateboarding is the co-ordination of the skater and his board, clearly defines the difference between the two sports, yet each are uniquely connected with a blending of technical perfection and overall athletic superiority. Akin to that, the biking world just blew up and what were once inconceivable aerials are now mandatory if you want to ascend.

Yet surfing gives as a unique insight into the sporting needs and development. Surfers must rely upon the capricious nature of weather acting upon the ocean to create, what amounts to a fleeting moment in time, a wave that allows an attempt at performing a specific maneuver. This amounted to roughly a 20-year gap in the time it took surfers to finally incorporate aerial maneuvers into the rhythm and flow of riding a wave. The fact that a skater can practice a trick over and over again took the sport from imitating surf style carving to teaching surfers the technical and physical approach needed to successfully perform tricks and aerial antics. In fact most, if not all of surfing's new school aerial enthusiasts, have a strong background in skateboarding.

Now the technical side of surfing has become glaringly apparent due to the almost gymnastic nature of the aerial maneuvers currently being attempted. The result of this phenomenon is the increased incidence of injuries to knees, ankles, and shoulders that could be prevented with a good training regime. But equally so it pointed out that for Surfing and the other sports to really blossom – training and preparation would be a part of the next evolution!

So basically, I've been involved with professional skateboarding, surfing and more recently wakeboarding as a commentator/participant/official since 1978. Of late my job as Head Judge for the Downhill Skateboarding and Street Luge events at the NBC Gravity Games in 99, 00, 01 and 02, brought me into the midst of the Extreme Sports scene. As an inside observer, I've had the opportunity to spend hours watching and analyzing the performances of the wide variety of competitors involved in all the sports presented. It has always been evident to me that on all performance levels, these athletes would totally benefit from augmenting their training with targeted strength, mobility and flexibility conditioning. I'm sure some do, but the question of proper guidance and accurate "coaching" from a qualified source made me wonder if such a person existed. I guess you might say that the question has been answered.

My first knowledge of Coach John Davies and his Renegade Training came when one of his devotees e-mailed me to ask about the application and specific advantages of Indo Board Balance Training in regards to traditional athletics. This prompted me to check out the Renegade Training web site thoroughly.

I was immediately intrigued by the directive Coach Davies issues to his followers: "Live The Code." This mantra is a strong statement requiring commitment and dedication to understanding a training methodology that operates well outside the confines of static gym workouts—where the focus seems to be more on getting buff and than based on a coach's understanding of what it feels like to paddle out or drop-in.

John's ideas on utilizing different yet innovative equipment made perfect sense to me and maybe, quite maybe, it was because in fact his Renegade approach was born in the surf or on a skateboard. The depth of these workouts covered such a broad spectrum of athletic endeavors that I made a note to investigate further. As so often happens, this was put off until out of the blue I received another e-mail from Coach Davies himself.

Remembering my initial interest I was stoked to be communicating directly with this apparently outspoken and controversial character, who so boldly presented himself as "Coach Davies." Once we got into our conversation it quickly became apparent that John and I had a great deal in common, along with a similar direction in wanting to enlighten the new genre of "Extreme Athlete" with a training program that specifically fit their out of the ordinary sports pursuits.

I thought it was a perfect connection between traditional sports and alternative sports because here was a guy who, sure, had trained champions at every level in football but grew up with a deep love and still to this day rips it up surfing or skateboarding daily just as if it was long-ago, back-in-the-day.

And so began our collaboration, from this great mutual respect, working toward the common goal of reaching extreme athletes who are interested in enhancing their performance to levels that no one has imagined. Coach Davies' dedication to teaching a sound program of using "out of the ordinary" training methods that are needed for the Extreme sports, will undoubtedly improve the athlete's abilities as well as reduce the incidence of injury. The paradigm has changed again as the Extreme athlete will now surge forward with an entire new level of athleticism.

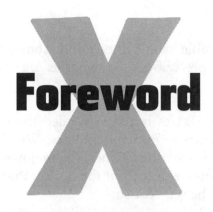

Foreword

By Grant Hansen

"Back in the day," as all us old-school guys like to say it, there was no terminology or classification to what we did. What we did was ride our bikes, skateboards, surfboards, etc., and had a blast, never imagining that we were paving a small road that would soon grow into a major highway for kids and adults who didn't relate to popular team sports. As a BMX racer and dabbler in freestyle (bike stunt) when the X Games (formerly called the Extreme Games) debuted around 8 years ago, the term "extreme" was used to "classify" what we did.

A few years later the terminology started to shift. Mountain climbers, skydivers, even matadors were thought to be the real extreme athletes as they defied death ... so we then evolved into "alternative sports". Well, that didn't last too long as our outcast behavior soon became one of America's biggest pastimes. So the term "action sports" became all the rage. What sport isn't an action sport??? I look back at the introduction of the term "extreme" and feel that although I've experienced riding my bike at 25 mph and coming to zero in an immediate rush of pain, I see how it's not that much different than catching a football in the open field only moments later to be clobbered by the free safety.

So what do we call ourselves? Well, how about athletes? But we really are a different breed of athlete. For BMX and skateboarding, there is no off-season. None. (I dare not leave out snowboard, ski, surf, etc., but these can be considered seasonal unless you travel the world or live in an area that offers the right climate year-round). Then again, there are some crazy, passionate souls who brave the sub-zero weather and hit the waves because the thrill far outweighs the stinging cold.

Extreme athletes are just that—athletes. But more often then not, extreme athletes only concentrate on skills training and not fitness training. High school and college ballers, track athletes, etc., often have the luxury of having a strength coach accessible (sometimes good, sometimes not worth the leg extension machine he prescribes). So what is the extreme athlete to do? Usually, they just ride.

The Renegade, Coach Davies has spearheaded the idea that proper sports-specific training is essential to extreme athletes. With the exception of BMX racers and a few riders of other disciplines, the majority of bicycle stunt riders, skateboarders, surfers, etc., suffer from the notion that riding and riding only is the answer to getting better. Not so.

Every athlete, whether your thing is football or local skate punk, needs to build what the Coach refers to as the "Wheel of Conditioning": skills, strength, power, speed, agility, balance, spirit. There are kids who go to the skateparks every day that possess some of these attributes, but think of it this way: you can catch more air if your can move more explosively; you can perform better aerials if your proprioreception is enhanced; and you can avoid injury with better balance, agility, stronger muscles and ligaments, and a refined focus.

I always knew off-bike training was important to my performance on the BMX track. It was my sprint training, rather than my skills, that helped me win the New Jersey State Championship a few years ago. But even at that time I didn't have a clue about what was really needed to train properly to win races.

As I learned more about the Renegade Training philosophies and protocols, I felt like I was winning a national title. I finally saw a proven plan of attack for the extreme world, not just the plan some of the most genetically-gifted (or drugged up) talents use. This is real training for real athletes. In this book you will learn all about Coach Davies' "Wheel of Conditioning," what it means to have the "Renegade Spirit," to "Live the Code," and to train with a relentless desire to be the best. If you follow the information in this book, you will pedal faster, jump farther, be better prepared for falls (prehab), and have a level of focus you've never imagined.

Too many kids (and adults) are lost behind the mesmerizing thumb tricks of home video games; too many kids are fattening up because they're riding around on motorized Gopeds, rather than pedaling a bike or pushing a skateboard; too many kids are embarrassed to take their shirt off at the beach and will never know the sweet sensation of getting to the impact zone and catching that wave.

Too many adults have played their way through high school and college and their athletic careers have all but ended because unless you're an elite athlete, the doors to football and other sports are all but closed; too many people confuse body building with athletic training; too many people see genetic wonders who'd probably succeed no matter what and they try to emulate them rather than seek out the truth. Renegade Training for Extreme Sports will raise as many questions as it answers, for the more you learn, the more you'll want to know.

Read the book carefully and go at your own pace. Step up to the challenge and never say die. As always, Live the Code and feel the flow.

Grant Hansen
Managing Director, Renegade Training International
Editor-in-Chief, BMXtreme.com

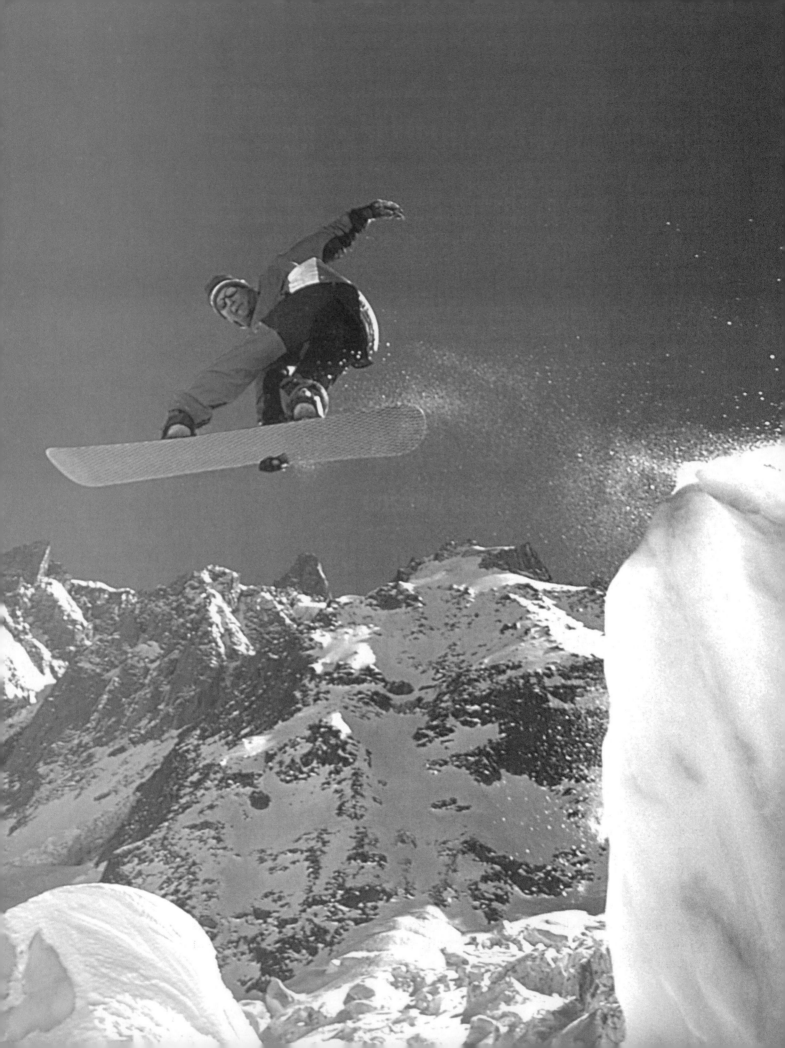

Introduction

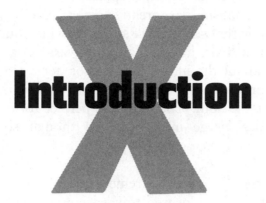

The so-called *Xtreme sports*—such as skateboarding, snowboarding, surfing, wakeboarding, BMXing, and mountain biking—have rightly gained in popularity over the last few decades. In fact, Xtreme sports (or *action sports*, as they are marketed now) have captivated participants worldwide, finding a following among those individuals who were not (or perhaps never were) satisfied by the status quo of more traditional team sports. And looking beyond the simple confines of traditional sporting pastimes has raised the bar of sports enjoyment and participation, prompting the introduction of new versions of these sports to the excitement of those who truly have a "feel" for the Xtreme. In fact, Xtreme sports have come to embody the present generation's sporting desire throughout the world.

Some may be surprised to learn that Xtreme sports have been around for 30 years or more. (Surfing, the original Xtreme sport, is even older than that!) The advent of skateboarding is generally considered the benchmark because when skateboarding burst on the scene, it quickly established itself as one of the most exciting and spectacular of all sports. Of course, right from the start, skateboarders abandoned conventional athletics and pushed the envelope of generally accepted activities. And while the legends of the early period—such as Stacy Peralta, Tony Alva, and, of course, Bones Brigade—weren't household names, as were other sports greats of the day, they were mega-icons to the original Xtreme devotees.

Without question, the subculture that grew up around skateboarding was a unique by-product—something that had never happened before. Perhaps this explains, in part, the negative, counter-culture image of the skateboarder that exists even today, to some extent. Sadly, few among the general public truly understand the extraordinarily positive influence that skateboarding has had. Top skateboarders like Andy MacDonald send a highly positive message about participation and comraderie to today's youths. I've worked in virtually every sport there is, and I dare say that few of them can hold up their top athletes as modeling such values! It's time for Xtreme sports to be accepted as the great influences they are.

Another positive aspect of Xtreme sports is that they are art forms—expressions of individualism, part creative genius mixed with a physical need to feel the rush. And in that sense, these sports provide boundless opportunities to express oneself, much like having a great canvass to paint or rock to sculpt. Xtreme sports are about the individual—his or her artistry on a board or a bike. They are the products of individuals' thirst to push the envelope of sport as well as manifest the soul. They are the perfect form of sport, in which artistry and athletics merge in a beautiful though sometimes aggressive juxtaposition.

Some of the sports considered Xtreme—for instance, skateboarding and snowboarding—seem mostly geared toward young male athletes. Even so, I believe these types of athletic endeavors constitute the final frontier of sports, where age and gender set no limits and sport is done for the pure and honest love of the game—the thrill of the grind, slash, and carve, part artistic genius mixed with a symbiotic need to feel the rush. Part of the success of Xtreme or action sports might lie in the greatest drawback of many traditional North American team sports, such as football and baseball, in which participation is generally limited to males in their early twenties and even younger.

The other neglected group of athletes that have found their niche in Xtreme sports is female athletes. More and more, Xtreme sports are becoming non–gender biased, something that is well overdue in athletics. The emerging role of the young female athlete in a variety of types of competition gives testimony to this trend. And so in addition to age, gender has been eliminated as a boundary on athletic performance.

From the time Xtreme sports first appeared on the athletic horizon, they have been part of my recreational lifestyle. Be it surfing or riding that sweet Powell deck, I've been into these sports for most of my life. And therein lies another aspect of the beauty of Xtreme sports: They can be actively enjoyed well into middle age (although some might argue with me on this point). For many athletes, myself included, the canvas of sport is how they paint the journey of life. And whatever sport they choose to pursue, they go at it with youthful enthusiasm, now and forever. In this respect, athletes are ageless.

So, when the opportunity came along to write a book on training for Xtreme sports, I jumped at it! And it was only natural for me to utilize some of my Renegade Training philosophies in preparing a program to train for these sports. Without question, the concept of "holding nothing back" in, say dropping-in on a vert ramp also suited the warrior attitude needed for success on the football field. So, incredibly, you might say that the relentless, attacking approach of athletes in football was predated and even generated by the "give it your all" attitude of the original Xtreme athletes. Thus, the Renegade soul was born!

Renegade Training is, in fact, a good match for Xtreme sports because one of the unique aspects of these sports is that they uncover an athlete that is completely Renegade. I have gone on record on many occasions to say that I don't necessarily identify with the concept of the genetically gifted athlete. In fact, however, many people do. From the dawn of time, society has admired feats of physical performance, and elite-level athletes have been accorded mythical status. Some even believe in a predisposition of genetic gifts, wherein greatness can be traced to a mysterious bloodline. This fascination over athletic ability also raises questions about nature versus nurture: Are true athletes born with special abilities, or do they develop those abilities through training and hard work?

For me, this debate is pointless. Being a Renegade is about what's in your heart. While it's true that genetic coding cannot be altered, hard work— sometimes, brutally hard work—can develop greatness in those who are willing to make the effort. For that reason, my greatest career goal as a coach and trainer has been to teach young athletes of seemingly common ability that greatness lies within each of them—and I have proven that with countless athletes. There are no limitations, no boundaries—just the individual and how good he or she wants to be.

This notion is the foundation of Renegade Training and its approach to developing athletes. For every individual, there is a *pathway to greatness* that, if followed, will lead the athlete toward his or her greatest goal. Success is simply the only option. It is a pattern of behavior. That pattern is not a circumstantial event but a well-orchestrated model. In terms of sports, triumph is not a haphazard result but the product of days of hard training and holding onto a "never say die" attitude.

Many athletes fail simply because they don't have a well-developed plan for achieving success. This is especially true in Xtreme sports, where the bar of performance is constantly being raised. It may be hard for some to admit, but the X-athlete is perhaps the most dedicated of all athletes. The commitment and dedication needed to learn street tricks—say, rippin' up the vert ramp, shredding a concrete pool in skateboarding, or performing incredible maneuvers in surfing—is extraordinary, and this learning often comes through tough and painful lessons. Few athletes in traditional sports exhibit the drive of Xtreme athletes like legendary BMX rider Mat Hoffman. While his commitment to excellence has resulted in some horrific injuries, he has taken BMX Vert to the astonishing level it is today.

Every X-athlete has known hard work and spent countless time and energy riding or climbing. Days of perfecting maneuvers have become weeks and years. Given this level of tenacity, performance in the Xtreme sports has improved at an alarming rate. Yet most X-athletes spend their time developing skills in what is termed in coaching circles sport-specific training, all the while ignoring the importance of developing themselves athletically to improve performance. In other words, the emphasis on skills has come at the complete expense of such physical factors as strength and conditioning.

When I've discussed training with top-level competitive surfers, bikers, and wake-, snow-, and skateboarders, they have told me that dry-land training is nearly impossible for them because they compete year-round. My response has been that they, like the great athletes of traditional sports, would find that as they improved athletic conditioning in a manner applicable to their sport, their sporting performance would go through the roof.

Quite simply, little or no information is available on how athletes in these sports should prepare beyond doing skill work. The effect of this information void is realized when X-athletes fail to meet their goals and become aware of their unrealized potential. At that point, the maddening question of "What if?" haunts them. Renegade Training can prevent that from happening by developing Xtreme athletes for which performance and thus victory are limitless. The goal of this book is to provide the specific tools needed to condition athletes so they can perform in sports—Xtreme sports as well as others—to the best of their ability.

The Renegade training philosophy is, in fact, rooted in the die-hard work ethic of a bygone era—one that will no doubt shock many of today's youth, whose low threshold of work capacity and laissez faire approach to physical development has made them seriously unfit. The X-athlete is a refreshing contradiction in that he or she genuinely enjoys physical activity and stays in general condition for his or her sport by practicing it endlessly.

For some, the notion of applying Renegade Training to the world of Xtreme sports is a little like supercharging the family SUV with racing fuel: way too scary to imagine but oh, so impossible to resist. So, be prepared! In taking Renegade Training to the Xtreme, I will bring action sports to an entirely new level. R

Chapter One

The Renegade Plan of Attack—What It Takes to Xcel as an Xtreme Athlete

To attack the future of sports—that, being Xtreme sports—requires thinking "outside the box" and examining every training element specifically in terms of these sports. This isn't about simple strength training and conditioning; rather, it's about what will make you better on the ramp, waves, slopes, or course. Your mandate is to improve performance, not simply to put up numbers in the training room. And to do that, you sure as heck better be out there, rippin' it up!

I understand firsthand what it takes to succeed in these sports because I have been out there! I've made many of these sports part of my everyday lifestyle. I've also made a career as a coach and trainer, taking a "no holds barred" approach that some people have found controversial. Granted, other Xtreme athletes and enthusiasts may have the technical expertise to be proficient at their given sport, but they are ill prepared from the standpoint of physical fitness. And that's probably why to date, there is no training program that focuses on the specific needs of the X-athlete.

Recognizing that void is what made me apply the principles of Renegade Training to Xtreme sports. The tough work ethic that's at the foundation of Renegade Training will help you develop superior athletic skills. And for those of you new to this world, let me say that you will rarely find sports that push the envelope of adrenaline like the Xtreme sports. There's nothing like dropping in on a vert ramp or paddling out among some serious waves to give you that rush!

Yet the focus of this program isn't just to make you look buff after finishing a solid session of training. Developing your body so that it's in harmony with your mind is another basic principle of Renegade Training. Doing so will help you "see" better into your sport and thus compete at a higher level. It will also help you develop an attitude that will leave you dissatisfied with anything other than success. Only those of you already in the world of Xtreme sports truly understand the intense level of focus and drive needed to perform at your highest level.

True athletic ability is a complex balance of numerous attributes, all equally important. Think of it like a wheel, the *wheel of conditioning,* with each spoke representing a specific ability. For maximum results, each ability must be carefully developed through specific work—hard work! In the Renegade approach, the skills that are developed to maximize athletic performance are as follows:

Renegade Training Wheel of Conditioning

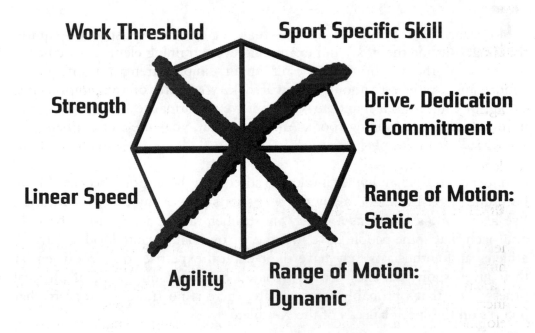

Work Threshold

Sport Specific Skill

Strength

Drive, Dedication & Commitment

Linear Speed

Range of Motion: Static

Agility

Range of Motion: Dynamic

• Range of motion:

There are two types of range of motion: static and dynamic. Whereas working on static range of motion is generally considered effective in injury prevention and rehabilitation, improving *dynamic* range of motion is chiefly directed at enhancing performance on the field of competition. The Renegade approach uses a variety of stretches—static and dynamic—that many trainees consider the most taxing portion of their development. This is more than just a stretching program!

• Agility:

To understand the value of agility, think about the very nature of Xtreme sports: Each is played within a tight environment using delicate maneuvers that are difficult to detect unless under the finite review of, say, a slow-motion video. Much of the agility work in the Renegade training program is directed at sport-specific movements, involving continual practice and refinement of individual maneuvers.

• Linear speed:

Having speed and being able to make explosive movements is a "calling card" of Renegade athletes. And while improvement in this area is often a by-product of training in other areas, such as strength and range of motion, it warrants a certain amount of attention all its own.

• Strength:

Given the many of forms of strength (such as speed strength, reactive strength, and absolute strength), this is an important athletic attribute. Renegade strength training uses hybrids of the classic Olympic lifts, along with some never before seen movements, to train the various parts of the body to work together in harmony.

• General Physical Preparation (GPP):

The concept of *General Physical Preparation* is at the core of Renegade training. In fact, it can be considered the foundation upon which all the other skill areas are built. As the name implies, GPP is an element of training that balances old-fashioned hard work with a variety of types of physical development, such as enhancing motor skills, increasing strength, improving muscular recovery, and promoting mental toughness.

• Specialized Physical Preparation (SPP):

As noted earlier, Xtreme sports are highly individualistic in the sense that each has its own moves, and Xtreme athletes have proven extraordinarily devoted to practicing these moves to the point of perfection. Renegade Training approaches this aspect of Xtreme sports through *Specialized Physical Preparation*, in which all training focuses on how to enhance performance in the particular sport, such that skills practice is woven into other types of training activities. But while you're preparing yourself to ride better, you still have to get out there and perfect your timing and movements.

In sum, this is the Renegade "plan of attack." It lays out the specific tasks that you must complete to improve performance, and it focuses your attention specifically on the job at hand. Thus, the mantra for Renegade training is "Form and function." Every task in your training must satisfy this mantra.

In addition to physical skill attributes identified in the "plan," let me reiterate the value of the mental attributes of *drive, dedication, and commitment.* They are quite possibly the real foundation of all training, yet they are often downplayed, particularly in current-day physical education programs. The truth is, however, that when athletes have to make tough choices about pushing themselves, the only place they can go for answers is to the proverbial "man in the mirror." Realizing the limitless power that comes with determination and focus is an important benefit of Renegade Training.

Chapter Two

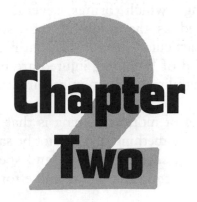

Xtending Your Moves— For Higher Performance, Less Fatigue, and Less Injury

Reading athletic training journals these days might leave you thoroughly confused about what the needs of an athlete are. According to these sources, it seems that the dedicated athlete merely needs to lift weights in order to improve his or her sports performance. But for those of us who have been around sports for most of our lives, this seems simplistic if not ridiculous. In training for the Xtreme sports, in particular, agility and flexibility seem key in being able to make the proper moves on a board or a bike.

Agility and flexibility are aspects of *range of motion*, one of the most important yet misunderstood and neglected areas of athletic development. Training to improve range of motion is often thought of as simply "stretching," implying that it's a passive activity and thus of limited value in terms of athletic development. Others would suggest that range of motion training has limited value because it's low impact and even tranquil at times.

This is all nonsense! In fact, training in this area requires hard work, total dedication, and a certain amount of pain or discomfort as you work to increase your range of motion. The bar is always being raised, in this respect, as the goal is to become more and more flexible. Many athletes consider this the most taxing portion of their training.

The major benefit of range of motion training is improved muscular harmony and motor functioning, which brings several more pluses. Physical performance is improved as the result of sport-specific range of motion training, which is of particular interest to X-athletes. In addition, muscle fatigue and the likelihood of becoming injured are both reduced; conversely, muscle recovery and rehabilitation from injury are improved.

A final benefit of range of motion training is that success is attainable for athletes of all skill levels—something that cannot be said about achieving goals in other areas of athletics, such as strength and speed. Enhancing range of motion has two simple determinants: desire and effort.

Clearly, an athlete's progress is impacted at every turn by his or her functional range of motion. Given this, the value of training in this area should never be doubted again.

How the Muscles Work

Before we get into the training, a quick overview of the basics of musculature is warranted. Muscles are composed of two types of fibers:

- **Extrafusal fibers** receive nerve impulses from the brain that cause the muscle to shorten and contract. The extrafusal fibers contain *myofibrals*, which contract, relax, and elongate the muscles.

- **Intrafusal fibers**, which run parallel to the extrafusal fibers, are the main stretch receptors. They receive messages from the brain that initiate a stretch reflex in the muscle.

Thus, each movement of a muscle is made in response to information from the central nervous system. The speed of these nerve impulses is intensified with improved range of motion, increasing the maximum speed of movement. This explains the improvement in muscle harmony and motor skills that comes from training in range of motion.

Improved range of motion also increases the supply of blood and nutrients to the joints, in part by increasing the supply of *synovial fluid*, which lubricates the joints. Having a broader range of motion allows the athlete to expel less energy in performing and decreases the likelihood of injury. For this reason, it's important for an athlete to warm up before performing. Think of it like bending iron, as if you are heating an object. Apply an easy, consistent tension to your muscles, and in time, you will become loose and pliable.

Types of Range of Motion

There are two types of range of motion, and both are vital to successful athletic performance:

- **Static range of motion** is enhanced by doing stretches and controlling muscular tension and breathing patterns. Tension is completely eliminated from the mind and the body, such that a relaxed sort of "zone" state is achieved.

- **Dynamic range of motion** is improved by doing activities that work specific muscles—for instance, running hurdles to work the hips. These activities are tailored to the athlete's given sport, such that they have sport-specific benefits.

Renegade Training works on both of these types of range of motion by using a variety of stretching activities, including both preworkout and postworkout routines. Much of the training is designed to enhance dynamic range of motion, such as doing hurdle/hip mobility work, tumbling movements, and weighted and nonweighted lifts.

Dynamic Range of Motion

Preworkout Stretching Routine

The Renegade preworkout stretching routine is designed to work on the functional aspects of the hips, improving joint mobility. While these exercises generally improve range of motion, they also provide sport-specific training for board sport athletes.

This preworkout routine uses a variety of the 10 hip mobility exercises listed below. During a typical workout, you should do 3 of these movements using a setup of 5 hurdles. Do 3 to 5 sets of each movement, and take minimal rest between sets.

Hip Mobility Exercises

1. Side Movement, Lead Leg Over
   (right leg from right side)

2. Side Movement Crossover Leg Over
   (right leg from left side)

3. Side Movement Alternate (from right side)

4. Front Movement From Side

5. Front Movement Down Center

6. Duck Under, Low Throughout

7. Duck Under, Pop Up Between

8. Duck Under, Twist, Low Throughout

9. Duck Under, Twist, Pop Up Between

10. Forward Zig-Zag, Duck Under

Note: The hurdles should be set at hip
height for all 10 exercises.

1. Side Movement, Lead Leg Over (right leg from right side):

Stand to the right side of the hurdles. Raise your lead leg over, maintaining a slight bend in the leg. Proceed to the next hurdle with a slight skip; be sure to stay on the balls of your feet as you plant each leg.

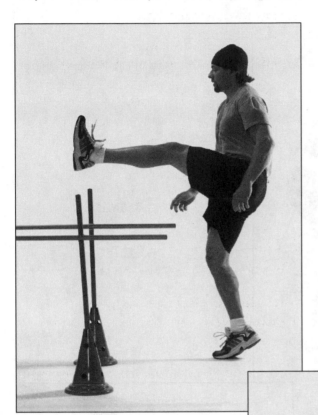

2. Side Movement Crossover Leg Over
(right leg from left side)

Stand to the left side of the hurdles. Raise your crossover leg over, maintaining a slight bend in the leg. Again, proceed to the next hurdle with a slight skip, and stay on the balls of your feet as you plant each leg.

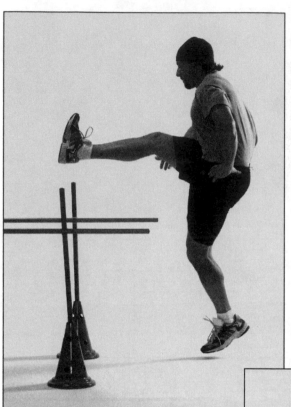

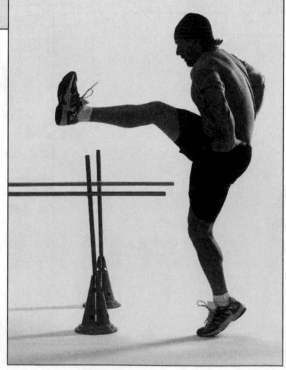

3. Side Movement Alternate (from right side)

Stand to the right side of hurdles. Raise your lead leg over (again, maintaining a slight bend) and then off to the side. Proceed to the next hurdle with a slight skip; stay on the balls of your feet.

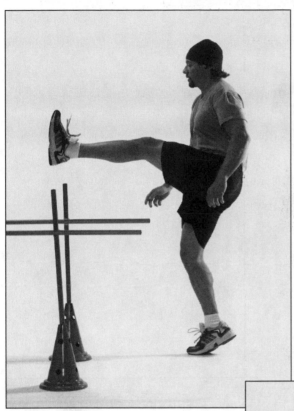

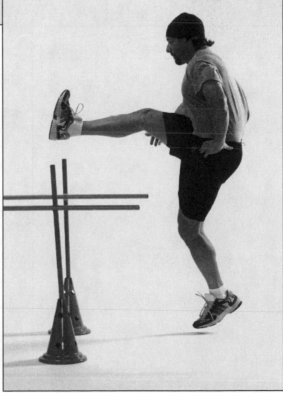

4. Front Movement From Side

Stand facing the hurdles. Proceed with one leg at a time by raising each knee over the first hurdle. Proceed to the next hurdle with a slight skip; stay on the balls of your feet as you plant each leg.

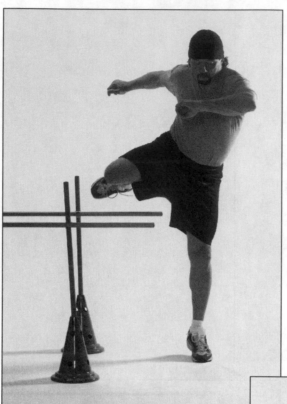

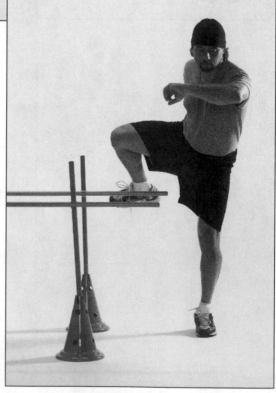

5. Front Movement Down Center

Stand facing the hurdles. Raise your lead leg over the first hurdle, and then bring your trail leg over the second hurdle. (The hurdles must be set close enough to accommodate this.) Stay on the balls of your feet.

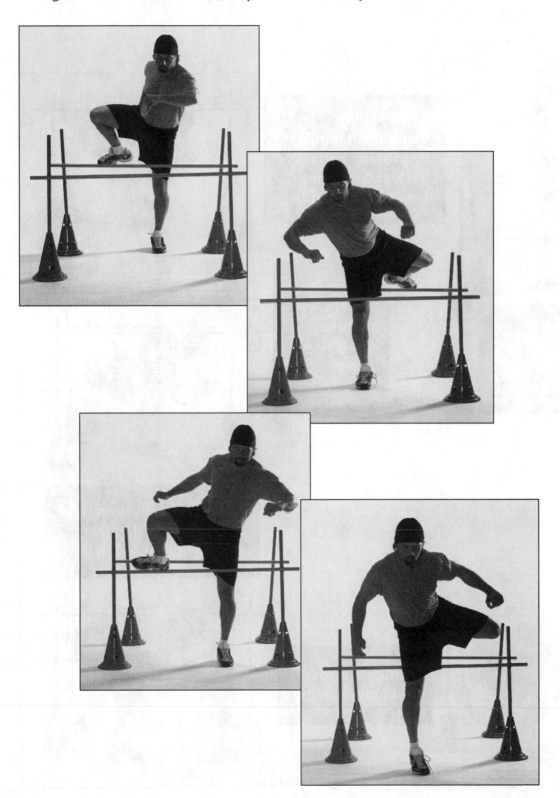

6. Duck Under, Low Throughout

Stand perpendicular to the hurdles. Duck under the first hurdle with your lead leg. Make sure your movement is initiated by pushing your buttocks back and that your feet always face forward. Stay in a low squat position throughout this drill.

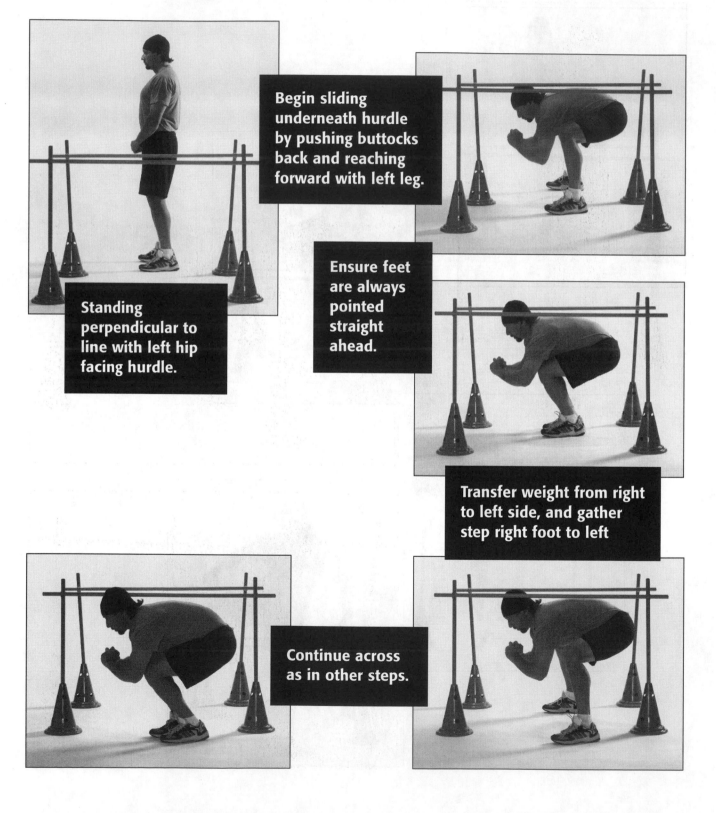

Begin sliding underneath hurdle by pushing buttocks back and reaching forward with left leg.

Standing perpendicular to line with left hip facing hurdle.

Ensure feet are always pointed straight ahead.

Transfer weight from right to left side, and gather step right foot to left

Continue across as in other steps.

6B. Duck Under, Low Throughout with Kettlebell

A tremendous option for advanced development of the duck-under is to perform while holding a kettlebell.

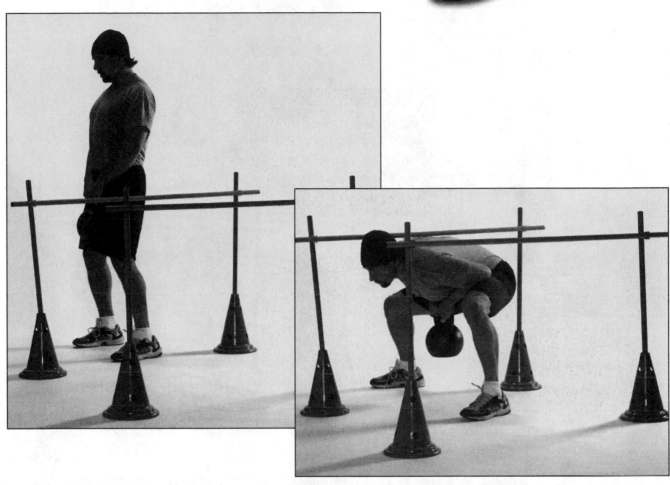

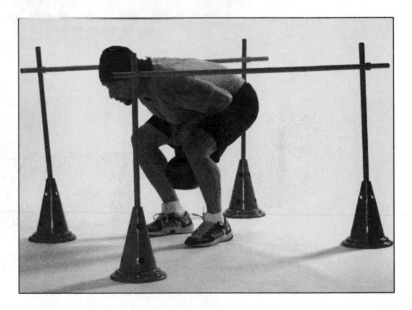

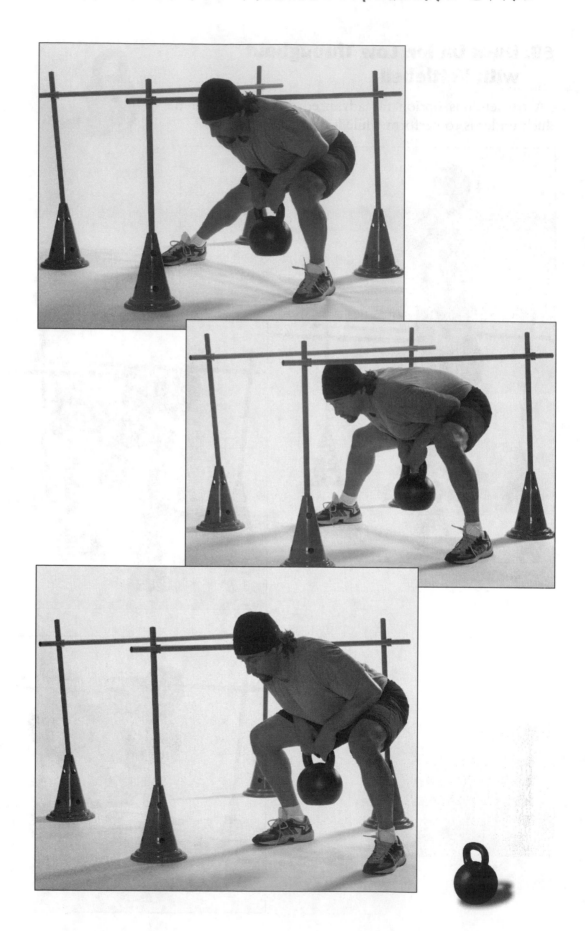

7. Duck Under, Pop Up Between

Stand perpendicular to the hurdles. Duck under the first hurdle with your lead leg. Make sure your movement is initiated by pushing your buttocks back and that your feet always face forward. Pop up from the squatting position after you clear each hurdle.

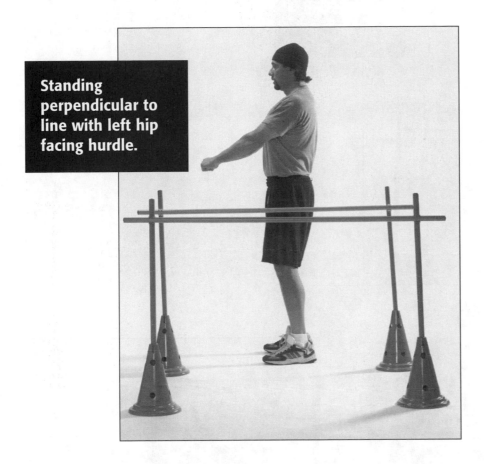

Standing perpendicular to line with left hip facing hurdle.

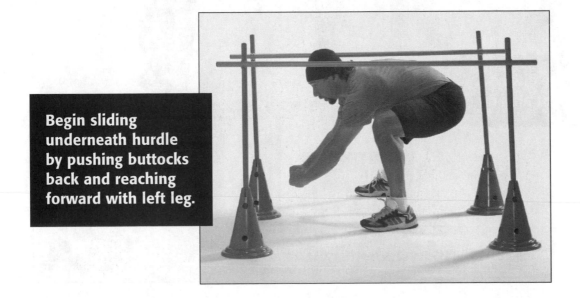

Begin sliding underneath hurdle by pushing buttocks back and reaching forward with left leg.

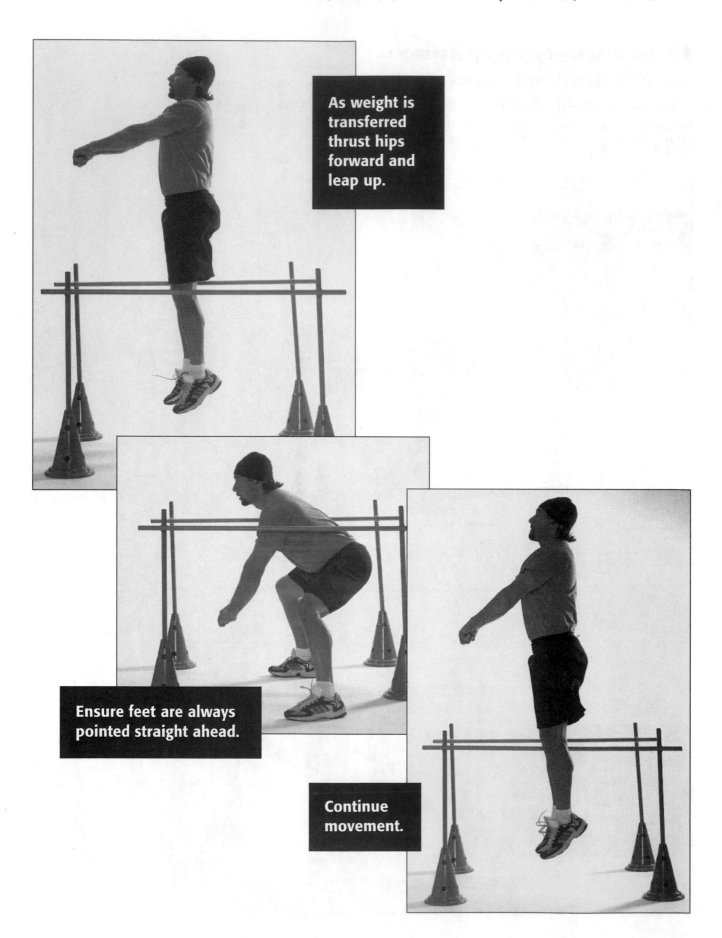

As weight is transferred thrust hips forward and leap up.

Ensure feet are always pointed straight ahead.

Continue movement.

7B. Duck Under, Pop Up Between
with Kettlebell

A tremendous option for advanced development of the duck-under, popup is to perform while holding a kettlebell.

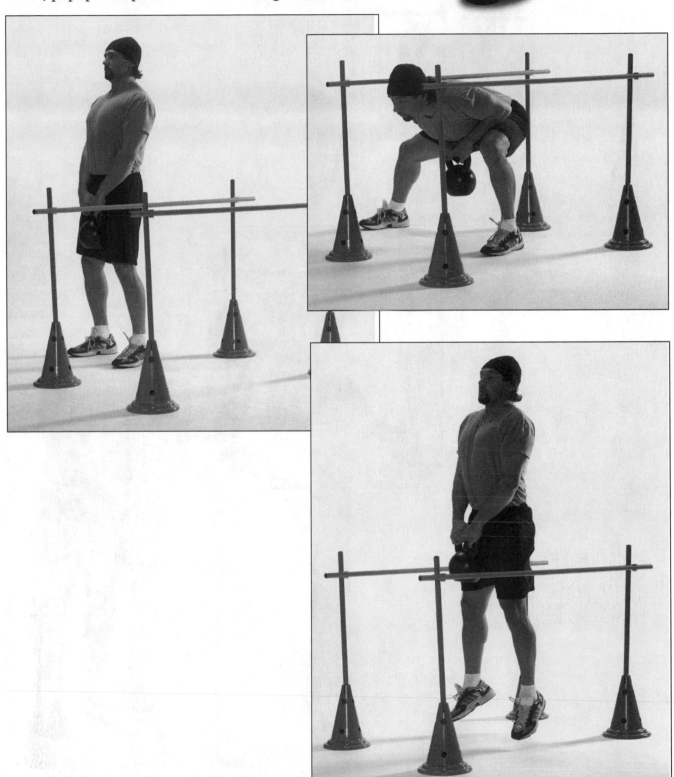

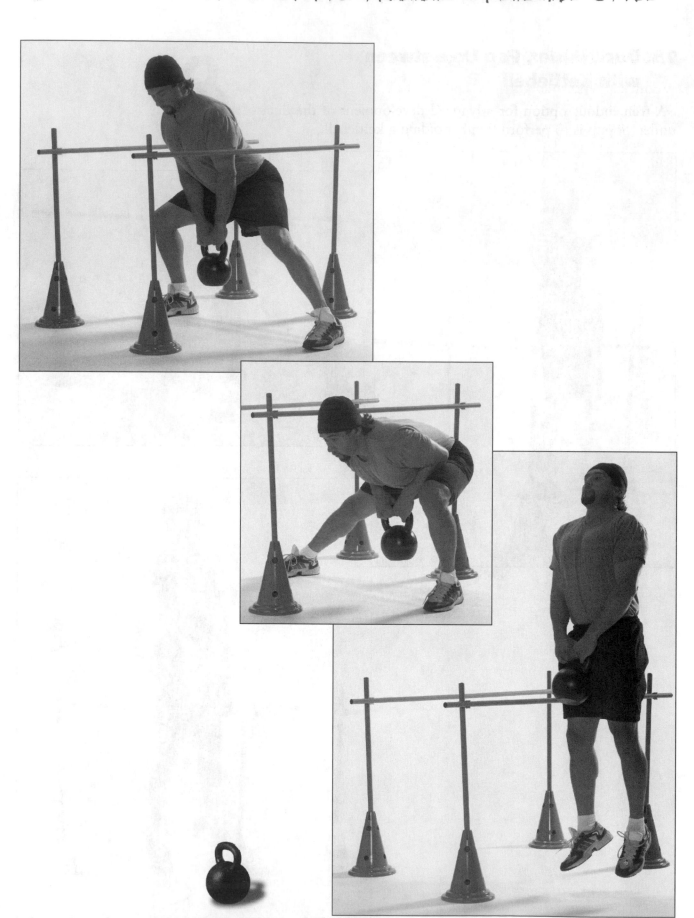

8. Duck Under, Twist, Low Throughout

Stand perpendicular to the hurdles. Duck under the first hurdle with your lead leg, and then twist to lead under the second hurdle with your opposite leg. Make sure your movement is initiated by pushing your buttocks back and that your feet always face forward. Stay in a low squat position throughout the drill.

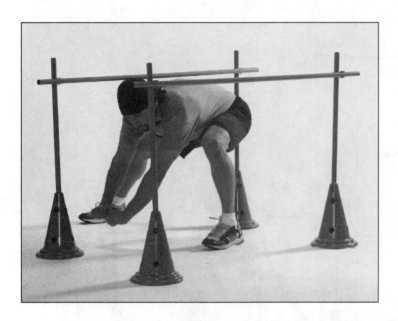

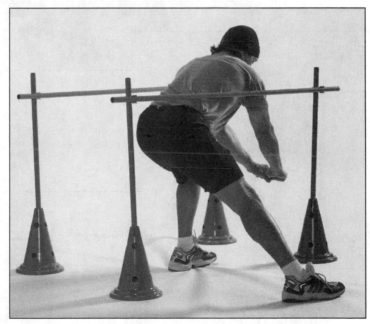

9. Duck Under, Twist, Pop Up Between

Stand perpendicular to the hurdles. Duck under the first hurdle with your lead leg, and then twist to lead under the second hurdle with your opposite leg. Make sure your movement is initiated by pushing your buttocks back and that your feet always face forward. Pop up from the squatting position after you clear each hurdle.

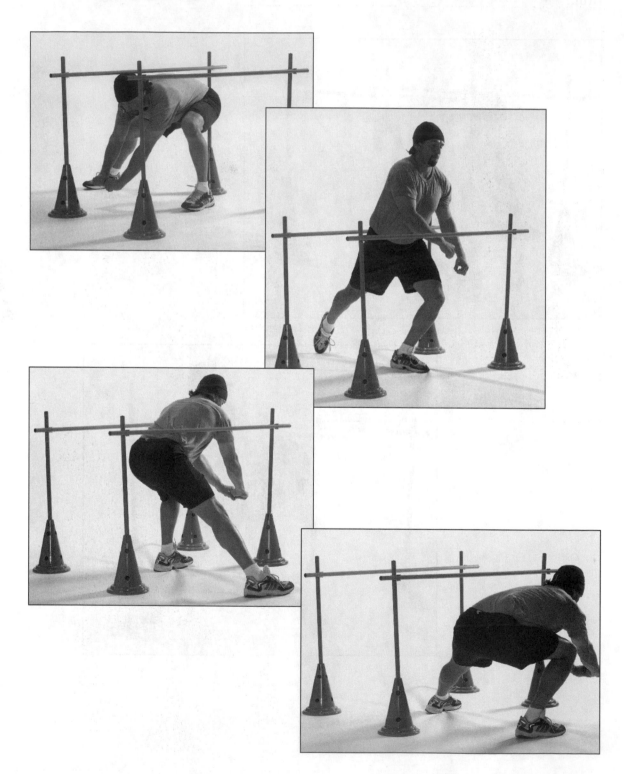

9B. Duck Under, Twist, Pop Up Between with Kettlebell

A tremendous option for advanced development of the duck-under, twist, popup is to perform while holding a kettlebell.

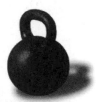

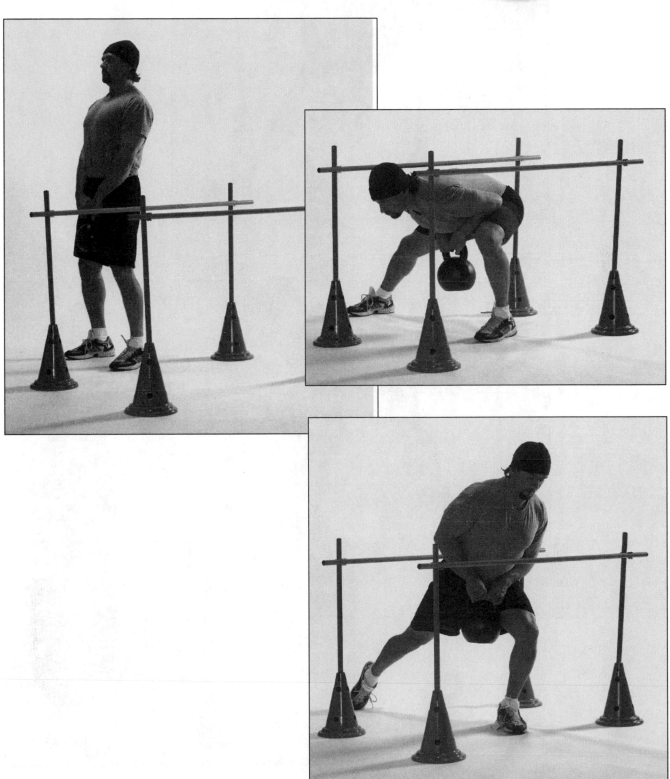

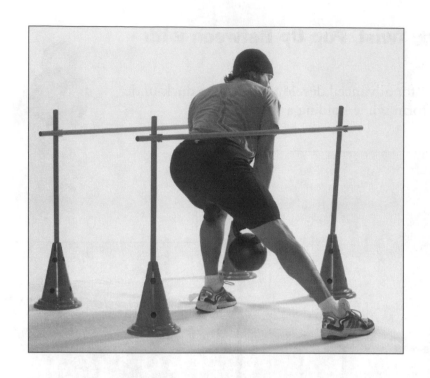

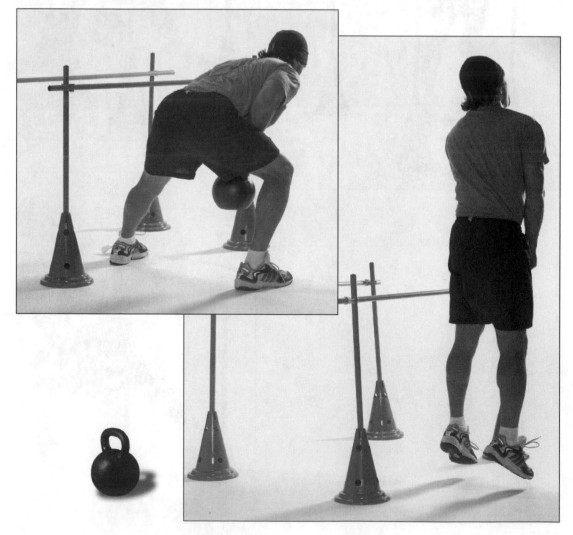

10. Forward Zig-Zag, Duck Under

Stand facing the hurdles, which are arranged in a zig-zag pattern, each successive hurdle offset one length from the previous hurdle. Duck under each hurdle, and pop up between them.

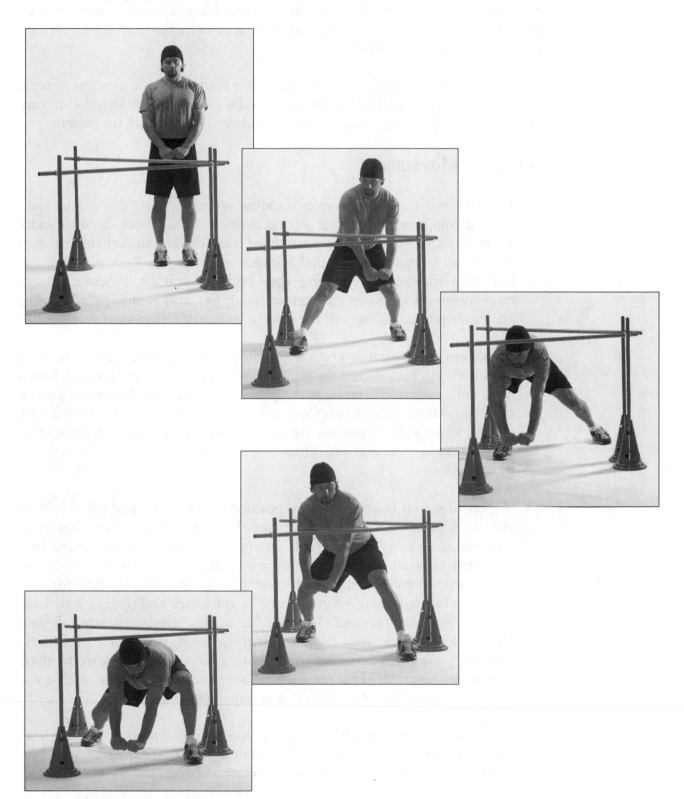

Tumbling

Tumbling is an extraordinary way to enhance total body harmony and kinetic awareness. When done as a warm-up activity on a daily basis, it can have enormous long-term benefits. By making tumbling a regular part of their training, many athletes have enhanced their range of motion and improved their general balance and control.

The tumbling movements outlined below are relatively basic in terms of what they involve and what they are intended to do. (They are not intended to turn you into a world-class gymnast!) You should do 3 sets of each movement.

Tumbling Movements

- **Forward roll to stand:** From a standing position, squat down and place both of your hands flat on the ground in front of you, about shoulder width apart. Tucking your chin to your chest, lean forward such that the top of your head contacts the ground between your hands. Push off gently to initiate a forward roll, curling your body as you go. Produce enough momentum so that you can get on your feet and return to a standing position upon completion of the roll.

- **Backward roll to stand:** From a standing position, squat down and arch your body backward until the top of your head contacts the ground. Reach back with your arms and place the palms of your hands flat on the ground on each side of your head. Push off gently to initiate a backward roll, curling your body as you go. Again, produce enough momentum so that you can get on your feet and return to a standing position upon completion of the roll.

- **Tripod to stand:** From a standing position, squat down and place both of your hands flat on the ground in front of you and about 2 or 3 feet apart (depending on what's comfortable for your size). Your arms should be bent such that your elbows are at 90 degree angles. Lean forward slowly and form a tripod by bringing your knees up on your elbows. Roll forward slightly while balancing yourself, curving your back and tipping your head until it touches the ground. To move out of this position, gently roll your hips back and bring your head up off the ground. Continue to roll back, bringing your knees down off your elbows and your feet back to the floor. As you roll back out of the tripod, generate enough momentum so that you can get on your feet and return to a standing position.

- **Spider lunge:** From a position in which you are on all fours but nearly lying on the ground, "climb" along the ground, keeping your body very low. (You are imitating a spider in this movement—hence, the name.)

1. Forward Roll to Stand

From a standing position, squat down and place both hands on the ground. Slowly roll forward and contact the ground with your head, tucking your chin to your chest and doing a somersault. Accelerate enough while doing the somersault so you have sufficient momentum to get on your feet and return to a standing position.

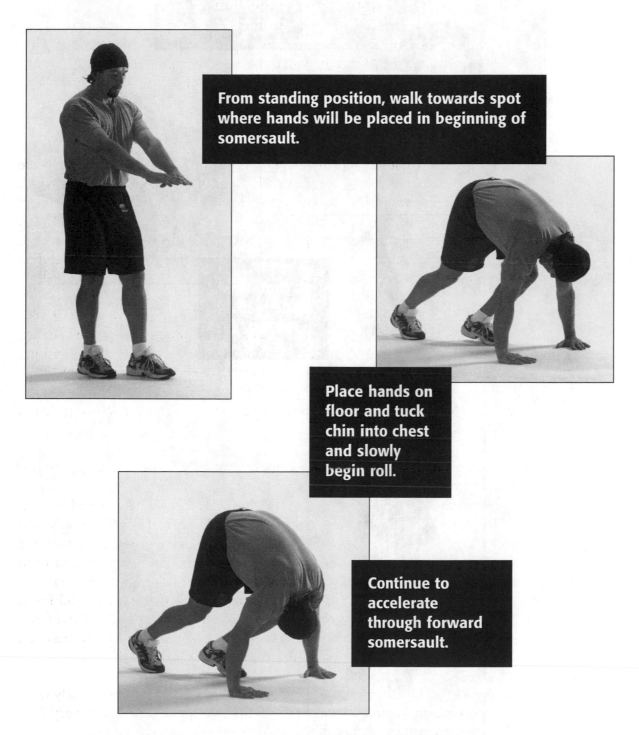

From standing position, walk towards spot where hands will be placed in beginning of somersault.

Place hands on floor and tuck chin into chest and slowly begin roll.

Continue to accelerate through forward somersault.

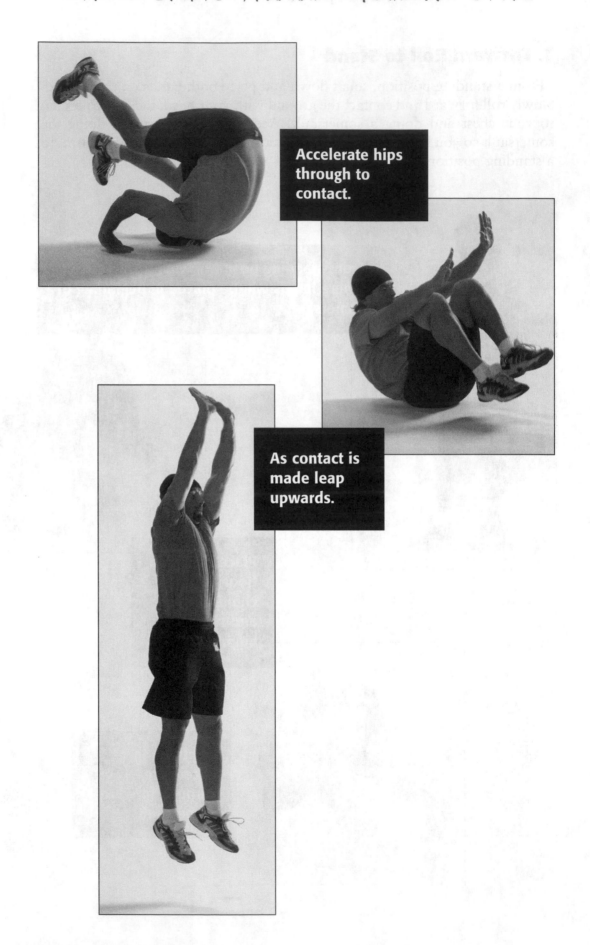

Accelerate hips through to contact.

As contact is made leap upwards.

2. Backward Roll to Stand

From a standing position, squat down and begin to roll backward. Place the palms of your hands on the ground behind your head, and as you begin to somersault backward, apply enough pressure to push off with your hands from the ground , get on your feet, and return to a standing position.

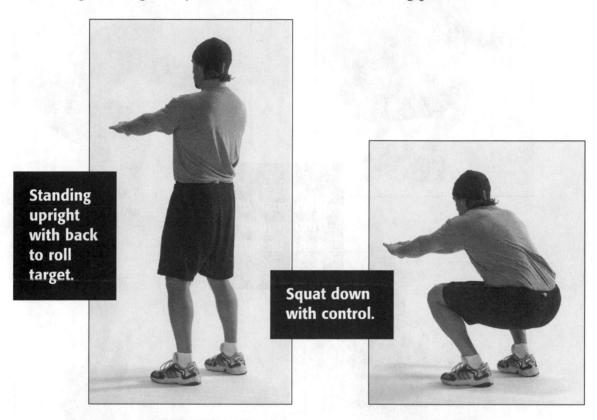

Standing upright with back to roll target.

Squat down with control.

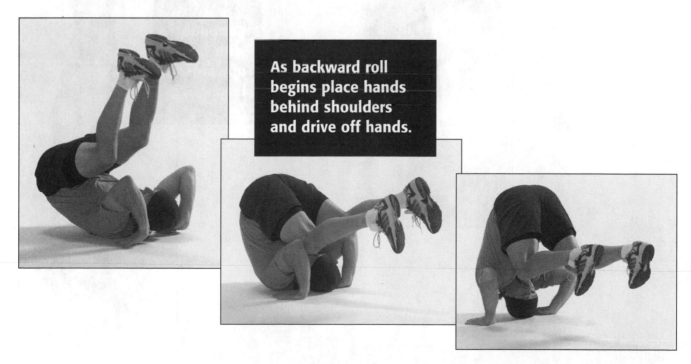

As backward roll begins place hands behind shoulders and drive off hands.

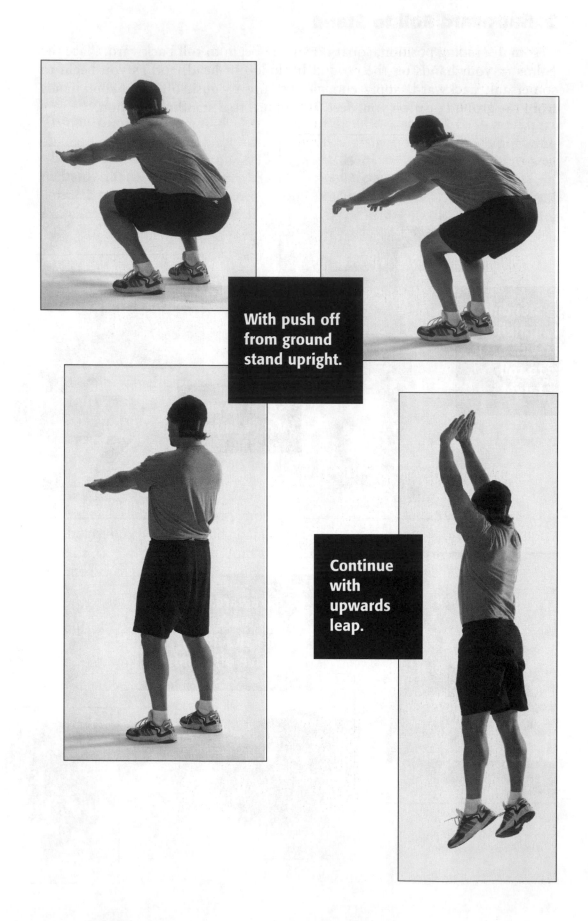

With push off from ground stand upright.

Continue with upwards leap.

3. Tripod to Stand

From a standing position, place both of your hands on the ground, shoulder-width apart. Squat down and form a tripod by bringing your knees up on your elbows. Roll forward slightly, curving your back and tipping your head to the ground. To move out of this position, gently roll your head back and up, straighten your back, and bring your legs down. As you roll out of the tripod, accelerate with your hips with enough momentum that you get on your feet and stand up.

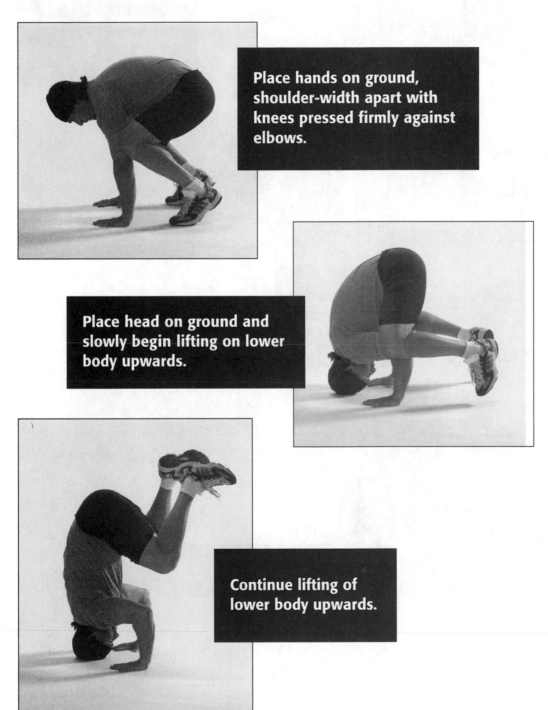

Place hands on ground, shoulder-width apart with knees pressed firmly against elbows.

Place head on ground and slowly begin lifting on lower body upwards.

Continue lifting of lower body upwards.

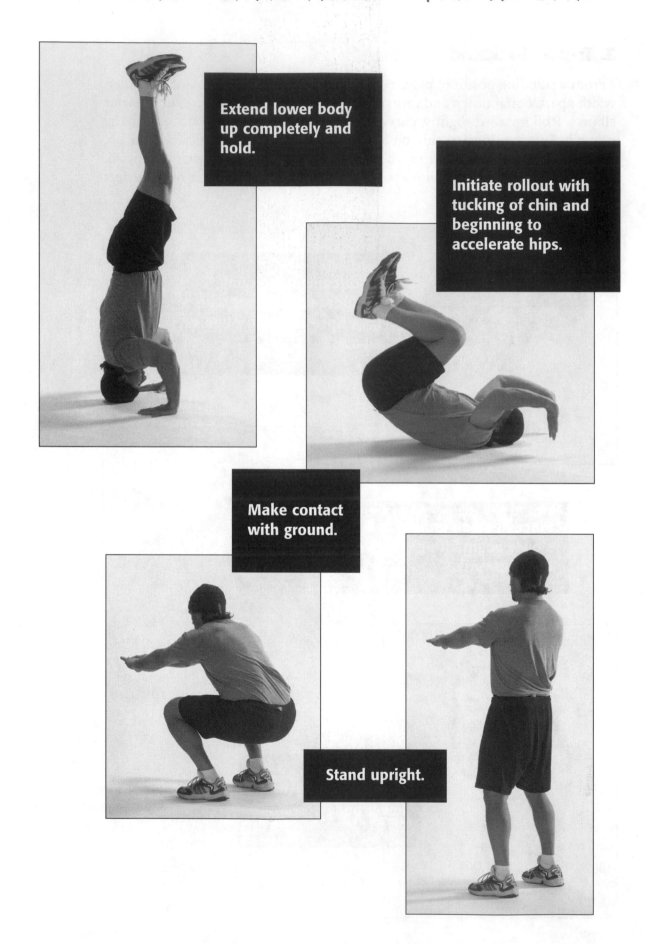

Extend lower body up completely and hold.

Initiate rollout with tucking of chin and beginning to accelerate hips.

Make contact with ground.

Stand upright.

4. Spider Lunge

From a position in which you are on all fours but nearly lying on the ground, "climb" along the ground, keeping your body very low. (You are imitating a spider in this movement—hence, the name.)

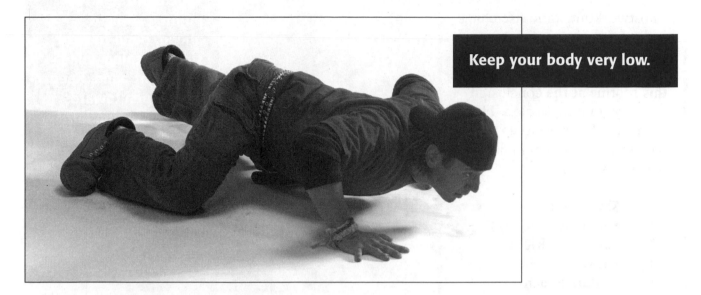

Keep your body very low.

Static Range of Motion

As mentioned earlier, training in static range of motion involves intense yet tranquil relaxation. Muscular tension and breathing patterns are both controlled while holding a stretch position. Tension should be completely eliminated from both the body and the mind, putting the individual in a sort of "zone" state.

The benefits of achieving this relaxed "zone" are especially value in athletic competition, when athletes want their actions to be reflexive in nature and not mired in thought and analysis. It makes sense that a more relaxed athlete will perform more to his or her ability, as well. No doubt, many great performers in the sporting world can relate to reaching this state, which can also be called "flow." In it, movement just happens in an instinctive and fluid fashion, without deliberate effort or purpose.

Given the extraordinary demands of Xtreme sports, *not* achieving the perfect concentration of the "zone" or the "flow" could not only destroy a performance but also bring disastrous results in terms of injury. As an X-athlete, it's imperative that you recognize this possibility and train to understand this deeper element of your cognitive processes. To help you do so, range of motion training has been woven throughout the entire fabric of Renegade Training. Look for it and become aware of your mindset and emotional state as you train.

Postworkout Stretching

Postworkout static stretching is done to enhance recovery using the stretches listed below. You should complete this routine at the conclusion of every training session. Hold each stretch for 30 to 45 seconds, and take minimal rest between stretches.

1.   Side Right
2.   Side Left
3.   Crossover Right
4.   Crossover Left
5.   Middle Reach
6.   Warrior Right
7.   Warrior Left
8.   Bent lunge Right
9.   Bent lunge Left
10. Triangle Right
11. Triangle Left
12. Standing Hamstring
13. Standing Twisting
     Torso Right
14. Standing Twisting
     Torso Left
15. Downward Dog
16. Cobra
17. Lower Back
18. Prayer Right
19. Prayer Left
20. Quad Right
21. Quad Left
22. Hurdle Right
23. Hurdle Left
24. Butterfly
25. Legs Apart Middle
26. Legs Apart Right
27. Legs Apart Left

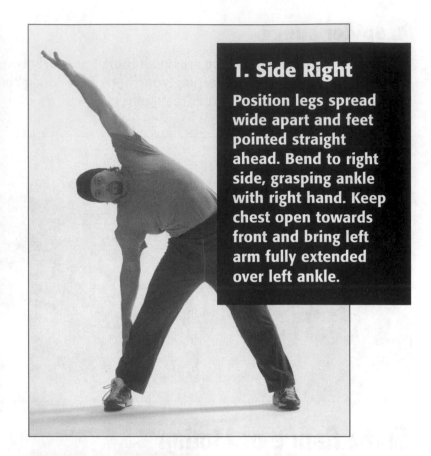

1. Side Right

Position legs spread wide apart and feet pointed straight ahead. Bend to right side, grasping ankle with right hand. Keep chest open towards front and bring left arm fully extended over left ankle.

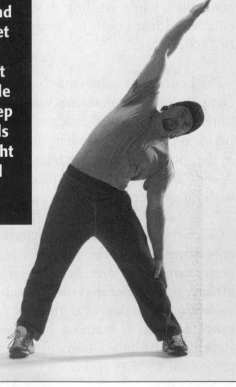

2. Side Left

Position legs spread wide apart and feet pointed straight ahead. Bend to left side, grasping ankle with left hand. Keep chest open towards front and bring right arm fully extended over left ankle.

3. Crossover Right

Position legs spread wide apart and feet pointed straight ahead. Bend over and twist to right side, touching left foot with right hand. Twist torso and open chest to left side and look above, extending left arm straight above.

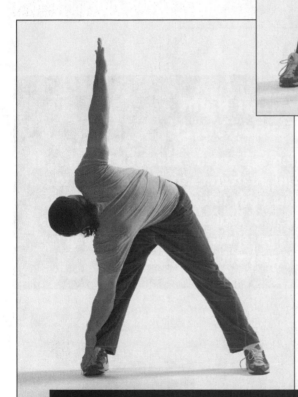

4. Crossover Left

Position legs spread wide apart and feet pointed straight ahead. Bend over and twist to left side, touching right foot with left hand. Twist torso and open chest to right side and look above, extending right arm straight above.

As left image but from side.

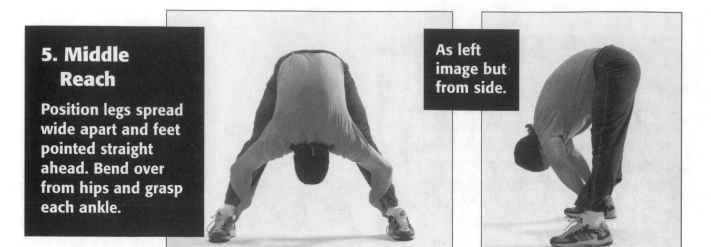

5. Middle Reach

Position legs spread wide apart and feet pointed straight ahead. Bend over from hips and grasp each ankle.

As left image but from side.

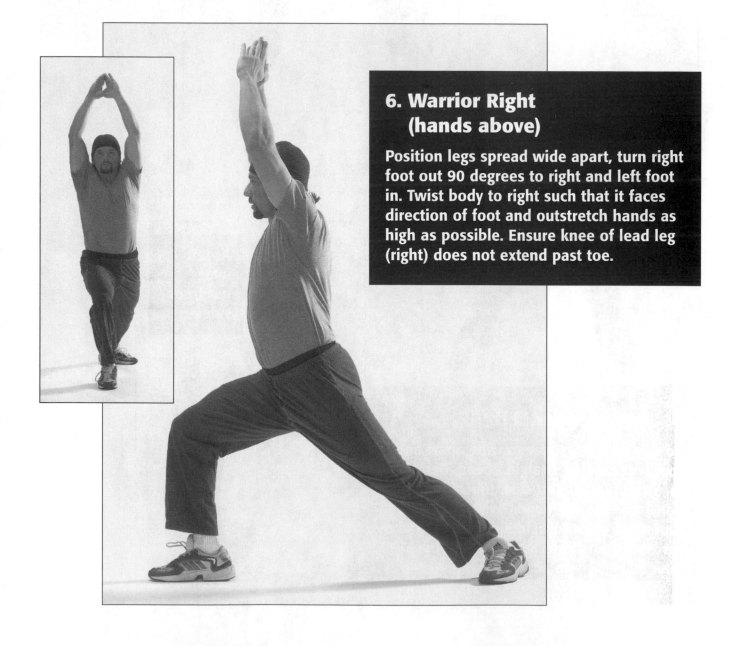

6. Warrior Right (hands above)

Position legs spread wide apart, turn right foot out 90 degrees to right and left foot in. Twist body to right such that it faces direction of foot and outstretch hands as high as possible. Ensure knee of lead leg (right) does not extend past toe.

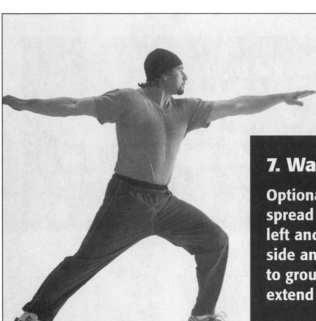

7. Warrior Left

Optional stance of "warrior" stretch. Position legs spread wide apart, turn left foot out 90 degrees to left and right foot in. Reach out with left arm to left side and right arm back, such that arms are parallel to ground. Ensure knee of lead leg (right) does not extend past toe.

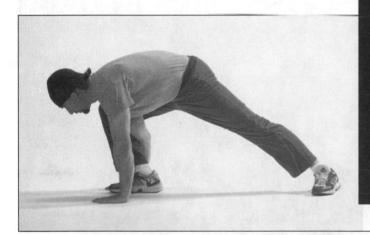

8. Bent Lunge Right

Position legs spread wide apart, turn right foot out 90 degrees to right and left foot in. Stretch down to right side and place right hand thru leg on ground to the right of the foot. Place left hand on ground directly across from right foot. Ensure back foot maintains full contact with ground.

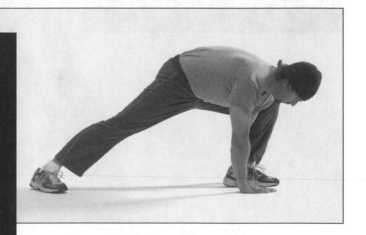

9. Bent Lunge Left

Position legs spread wide apart, turn left foot out 90 degrees to left and right foot in. Stretch down to left side and place left hand thru leg on ground to the left of the foot. Place right hand on ground directly across from left foot. Ensure back foot maintains full contact with ground.

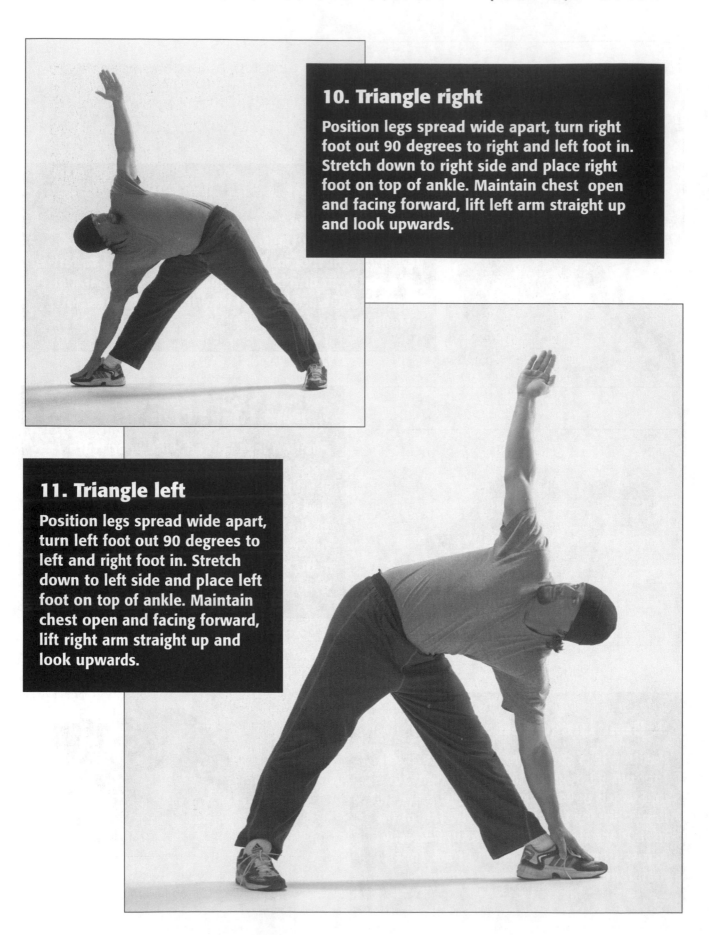

10. Triangle right

Position legs spread wide apart, turn right foot out 90 degrees to right and left foot in. Stretch down to right side and place right foot on top of ankle. Maintain chest open and facing forward, lift left arm straight up and look upwards.

11. Triangle left

Position legs spread wide apart, turn left foot out 90 degrees to left and right foot in. Stretch down to left side and place left foot on top of ankle. Maintain chest open and facing forward, lift right arm straight up and look upwards.

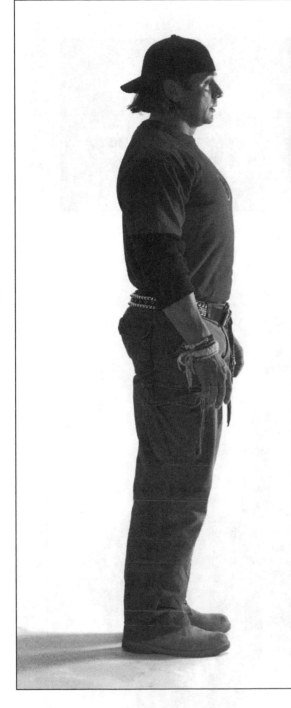

12. Standing Hamstring

With good posture pivot at hips keeping legs straight and rest hands on feet as if tailbone is being extended up.

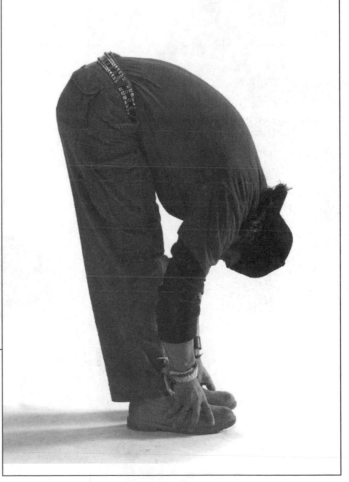

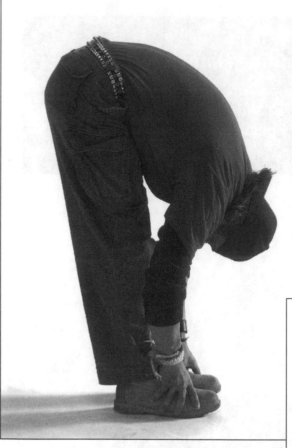

13. Standing Twisting Torso Right

From above position, push left knee forward, twist to the right and place left hand on right foot.

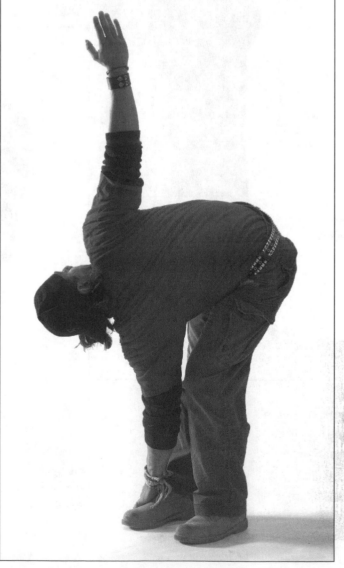

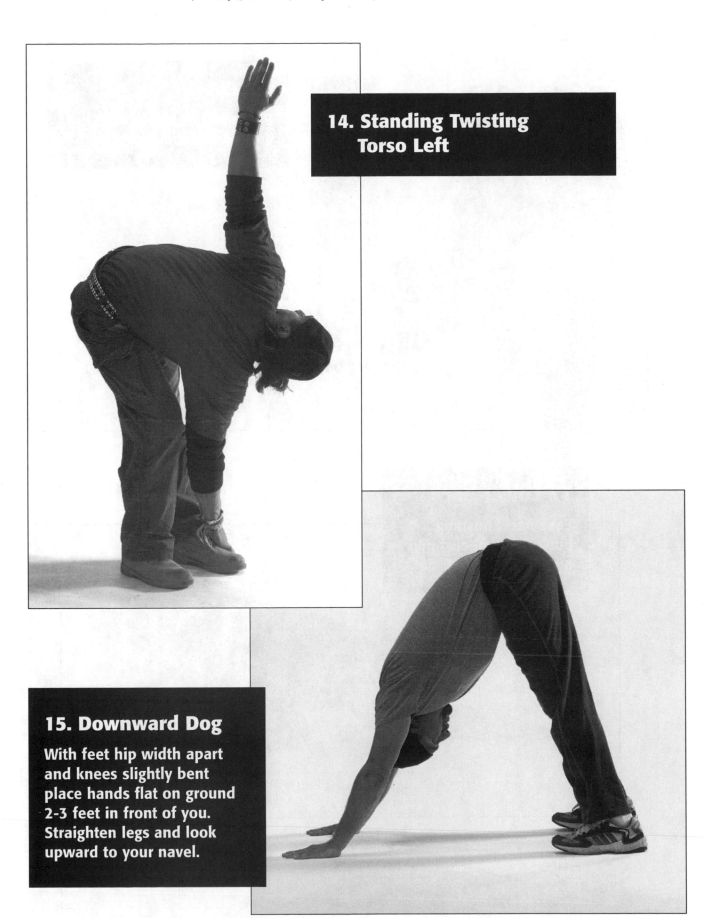

14. Standing Twisting Torso Left

15. Downward Dog

With feet hip width apart and knees slightly bent place hands flat on ground 2-3 feet in front of you. Straighten legs and look upward to your navel.

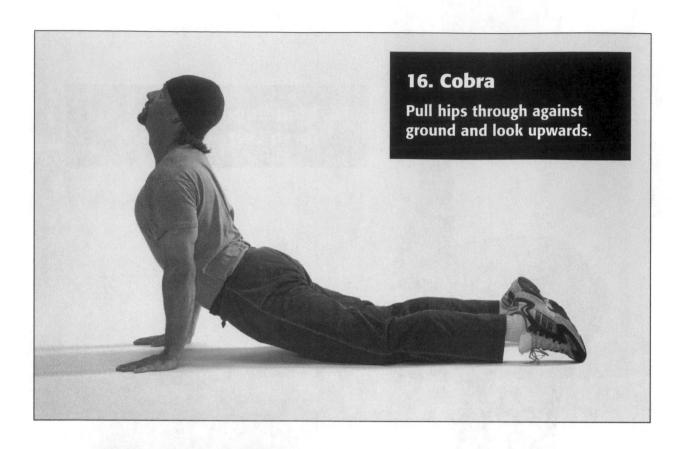

16. Cobra
Pull hips through against ground and look upwards.

17. Lower Back
Ease back, pushing buttocks to heels and arms outstretched flat.

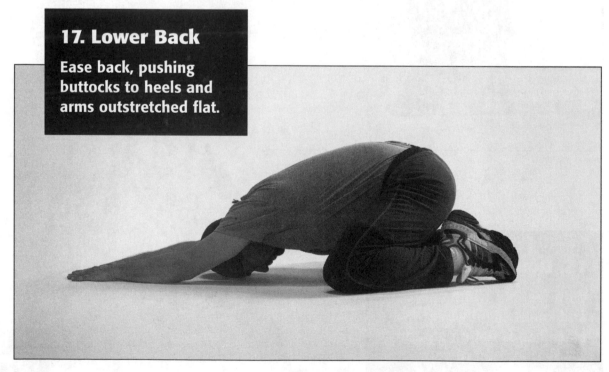

18. Prayer Right

Laying on ground, place right knee under chest and fold shin across. Keep back leg straight and reach arms outward with back as flat as possible.

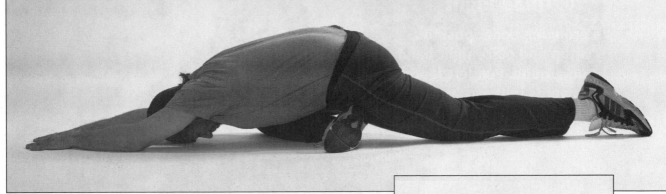

Front angle of stretch.

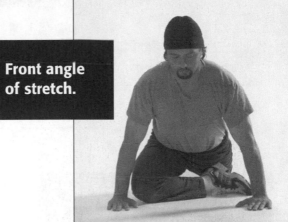

19. Prayer Left

Laying on ground, place left knee under chest and fold shin across. Keep back leg straight and reach arms outward with back as flat as possible.

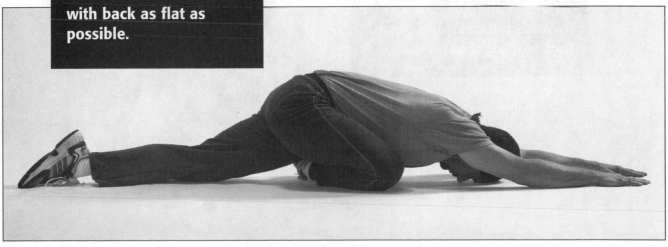

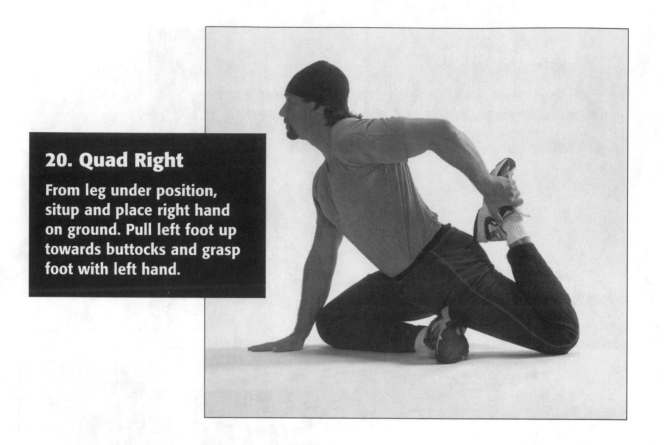

20. Quad Right

From leg under position, situp and place right hand on ground. Pull left foot up towards buttocks and grasp foot with left hand.

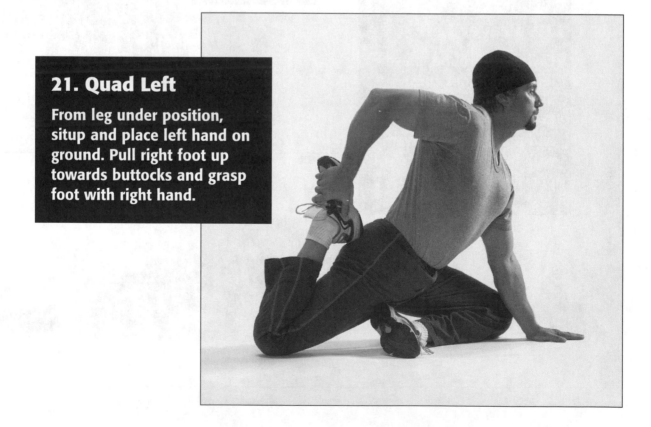

21. Quad Left

From leg under position, situp and place left hand on ground. Pull right foot up towards buttocks and grasp foot with right hand.

23. Hurdle Right

Outstretch right leg, with left foot against right thigh. Sit forward bending from the hip and grasp outside of right foot with right hand and inside of foot with left hand. Ensure shoulders are straight ahead and do not twist.

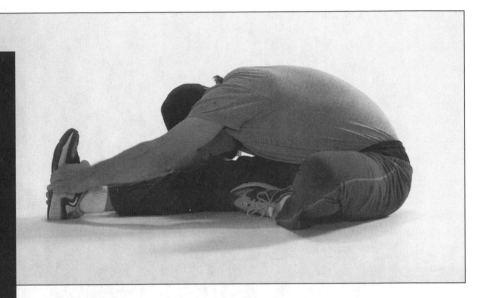

24. Hurdle Left

Outstretch left leg, with right foot against left thigh. Sit forward bending from the hip and grasp outside of left foot with left hand and inside of foot with right hand. Ensure shoulders are straight ahead and do not twist.

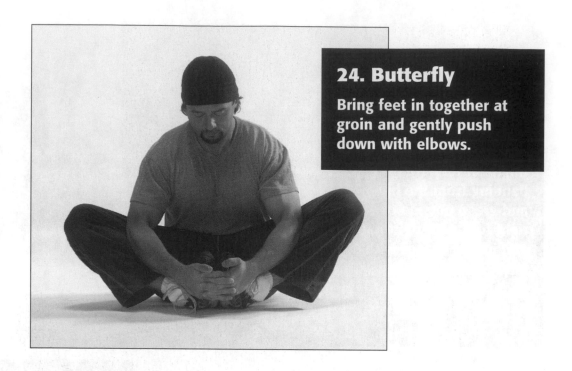

24. Butterfly

Bring feet in together at groin and gently push down with elbows.

25. Legs Apart Middle

Legs wide apart with toes pointed upward, ensuring feet don't roll outside. Sit forward by bending from the hip and grasp feet with respective hands.

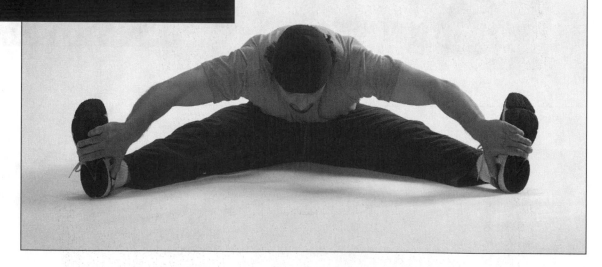

26. Legs Apart Right

Legs wide apart with toes pointed upward, ensuring feet don't roll outside. Sit forward by bending from the hip and grasp right foot with right hand and left hand on inside of right ankle.

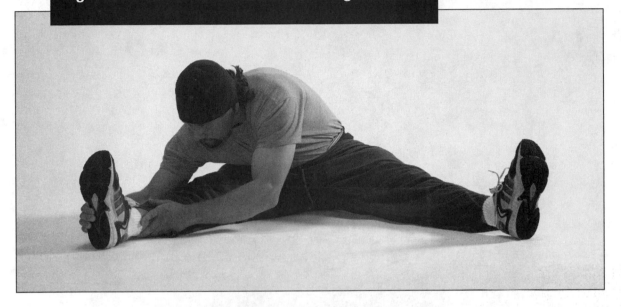

27. Legs Apart Left

Legs wide apart with toes pointed upward, ensuring feet don't roll outside. Sit forward by bending from the hip and grasp left foot with left hand and right hand on inside of left ankle.

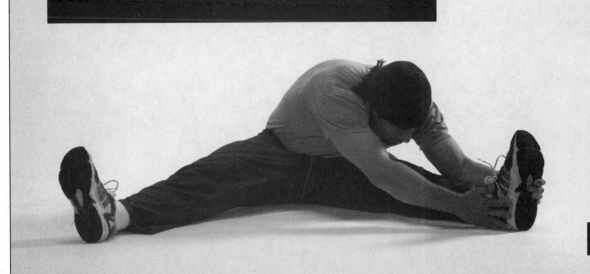

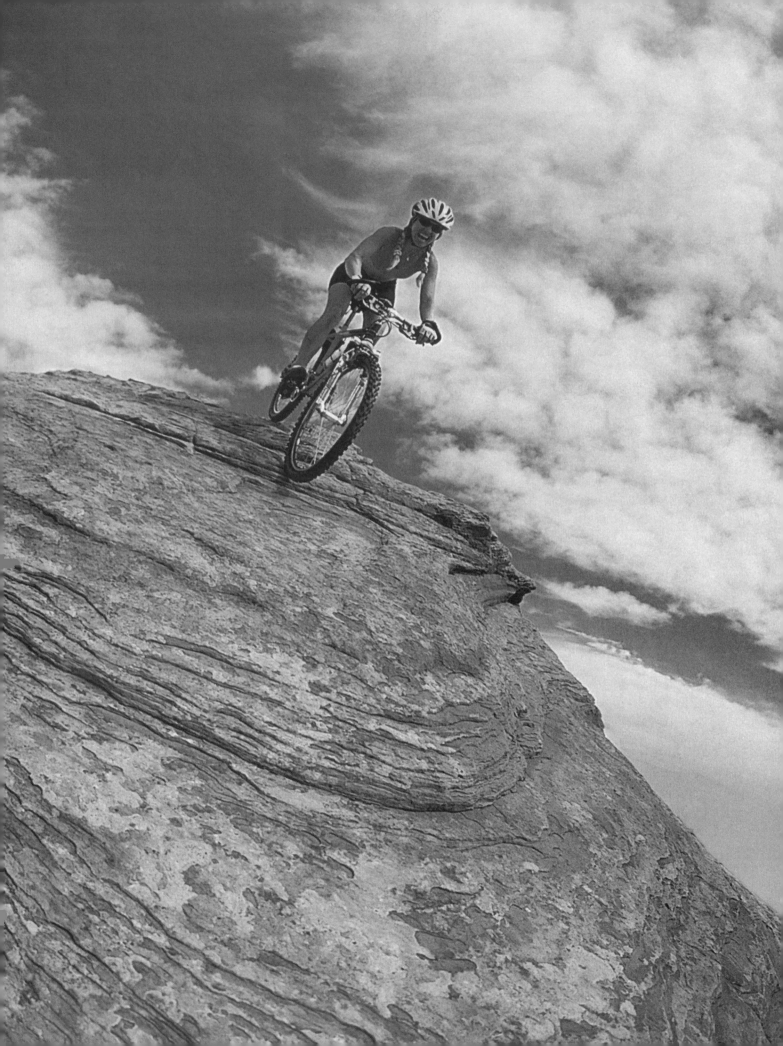

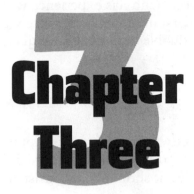

Chapter Three

Xtreme Agility—How to Achieve Cat–Like Balance and Super–Quick Reaction Times

In most Xtreme sports, success is determined by the execution of small, precise movements. So in addition to learning sport-specific skills, improving agility is extremely important for the X-athlete. The merits of agility training, which include improving balance and reaction time, are tremendous and will have an immediate and direct impact on performance.

The Renegade "plan of attack" takes an approach to agility training that also ties in with *Specialized Physical Preparation (SPP)*, which is the focus of Chapter 7. For now, let me say that in training for Xtreme sports, it is next to impossible to differentiate between agility and sport-specific skills. (This is clearly not the case in training for traditional sports, like football and baseball, in which the two have distinct drills and purposes.) Given this overlap, the training in this chapter is actually a combination of dry-land/quasi-SPP and agility, in which you practice movements similar to, say, a heel kick but in a manner off a board. The program uses a hybrid of rope skipping and balance work.

The Renegade approach to balance work, which uses Swiss balls and a highly specialized balance board, is somewhat controversial within the scientific strength and conditioning community. The fact is, however, that much of this controversy comes from *outside* the realm of Xtreme sports, and as I've already mentioned, the needs of traditional athletes are very different from those of X-treme athletes, particularly in terms of strength enhancement. (More on this later!) Anyone who has experience with surfing, snowboarding, or skateboarding will understand that the balance work done with Swiss balls and balance boards is invaluable because it is uniquely similar to the real sport.

Rope Skipping

The first phase of all agility training is rope skipping, which should come as no surprise. The history of rope work is steeped in tradition, and given the range of benefits it provides, it should be a consistent component of all future training.

Rope work develops a whole range of physical attributes, producing these benefits:

- Improved foot speed and hand speed
- Improved cardiovascular efficiency
- Enhanced motor skills/muscular harmony
- Reduction of body fat
- Strengthening of soft tissues
- Improved balance
- Increased work capacity

And along with these physical benefits, rope work develops the mental attributes of concentration and timing. Plus, skipping rope is relatively easy to learn, fully transportable, and inexpensive. Athletes of all levels can benefit from rope work.

Just keep in mind that in Renegade Training, rope skipping is not like the childhood game. It's done at a torrid pace and requires extreme focus. So be prepared!

The Basics of Rope Work

To begin, you need to consider the proper mechanics of rope work. Luckily, learning to skip rope is pretty simple, so your skills will develop quickly. Even so, you should start your rope routine at a moderate level and build up using an easy but consistent pace. Use *time* as your base in measuring your work. Consider the first few weeks of rope training as a phasing in to the real program. Your body will quickly adapt to the demands you make of it, and you will be able to attack this pursuit with ferocity.

There's no need to purchase an expensive jump rope; I tend to prefer the inexpensive plastic models, which can be easily adjusted. In selecting a rope or adjusting its length, make sure it's long enough so that when it's looped under your feet, it will reach chest height.

There are several ways to position your hands when jumping rope, and they offer drastic differences in terms of physical benefits. The most common position is to drop your hands naturally to your sides, such that the speed of the rope relies mostly on your wrist movement. This is a solid way to perform skipping.

An alternative hand position offers some interesting benefits for bicep development and also enhances foot speed. Instead of allowing your hands to drop, bend your arms up at 90 degree angles and pinch your elbows into your sides, such that your forearms are roughly parallel to the ground. Spinning the rope in this position will really involve your biceps and forearms, and once you adapt to this style, you will notice a radical increase in the speed of the rope.

Whatever hand position you use, you'll find that the speed of the rope will increase significantly as your skill level improves. A generally acceptable speed range for skipping rope is 90 to 120 revolutions per minute.

Movement Patterns

As you gain skill and confidence, you will want to

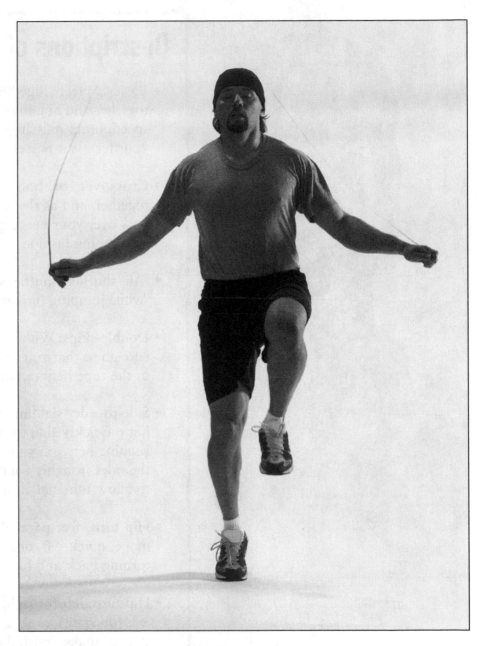

implement patterns of movement in your rope work. You can perform a virtually endless array of combinations, and you can always experiment. But the Renegade approach uses a simple pattern of movements in its total rope routine.

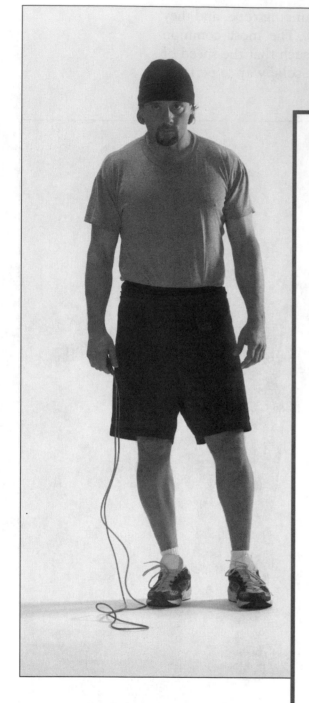

Descriptions of Sequence Drills

- **Basic 2 feet together:** Jump with your feet together and at a maximal pace; to increase your speed, jump only high enough so the rope clears your feet as it passes underneath you.

- **Crossover of hands:** Jump with your feet together, and as the rope comes up and starts to pass over your head, quickly cross your hands in a whipping fashion.

- **Ali shuffle:** Shuffle your feet back and forth while jumping (imitating the legendary boxer).

- **Double-skips:** With your feet together, jump high enough so that you can complete two revolutions of the rope between jumps.

- **Side-to-side slalom:** With your feet together, jump quickly side to side over an imaginary line running between your legs. Make small jumps to the sides (roughly 6 inches) and only high enough to allow minimal clearance of the rope.

- **Hip turn, feet parallel:** With your feet together, make quick 90 degree turns with your hips, turning back and forth.

- **Hip turn, left (or right) foot forward:** With your left (or right) foot in front, akin to a boxer's stance, make quick 90 degree turns with your hips, turning back and forth.

- **High knees:** Starting with your feet together, run in place, keeping your knees high.

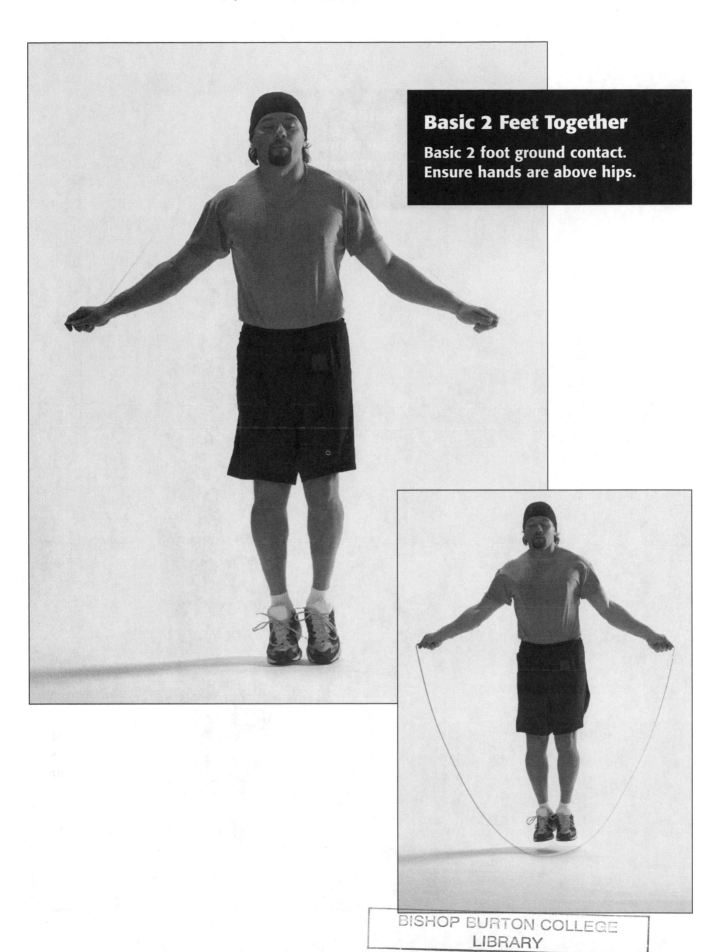

Basic 2 Feet Together

Basic 2 foot ground contact.
Ensure hands are above hips.

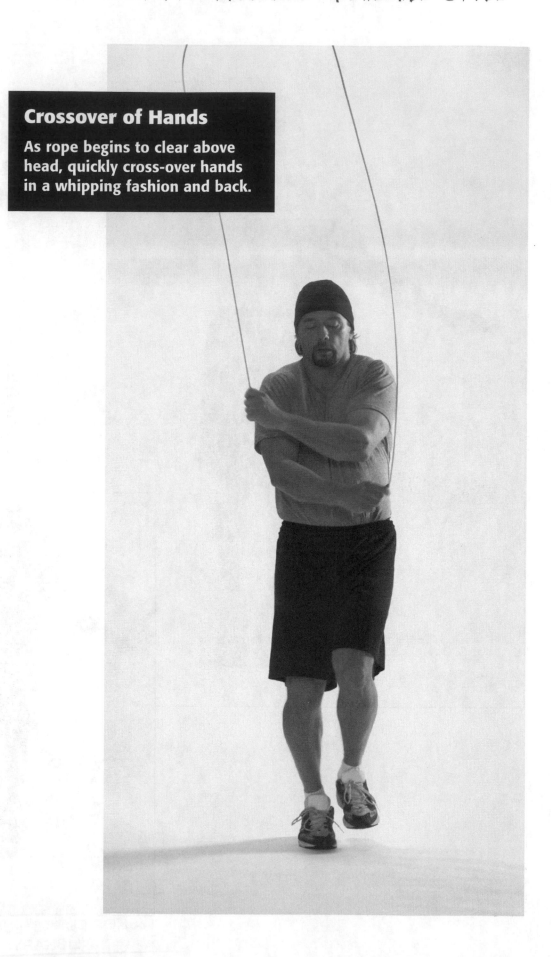

Crossover of Hands

As rope begins to clear above head, quickly cross-over hands in a whipping fashion and back.

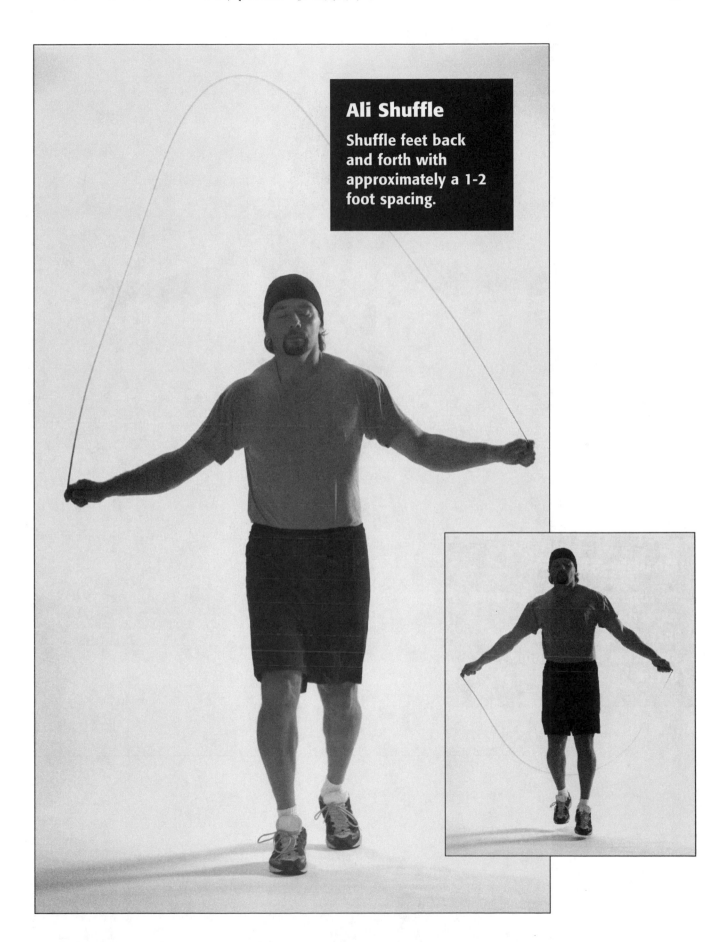

Ali Shuffle

Shuffle feet back and forth with approximately a 1-2 foot spacing.

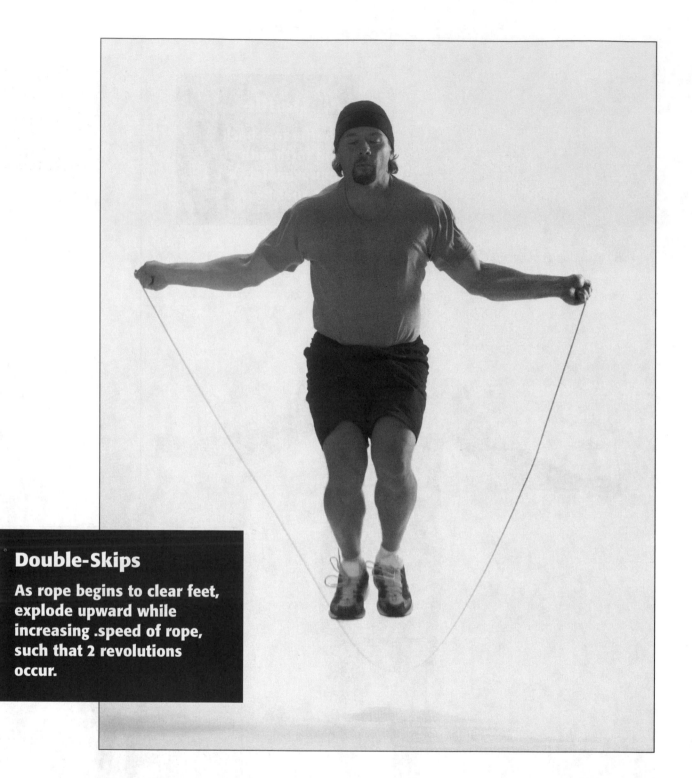

Double-Skips

As rope begins to clear feet, explode upward while increasing .speed of rope, such that 2 revolutions occur.

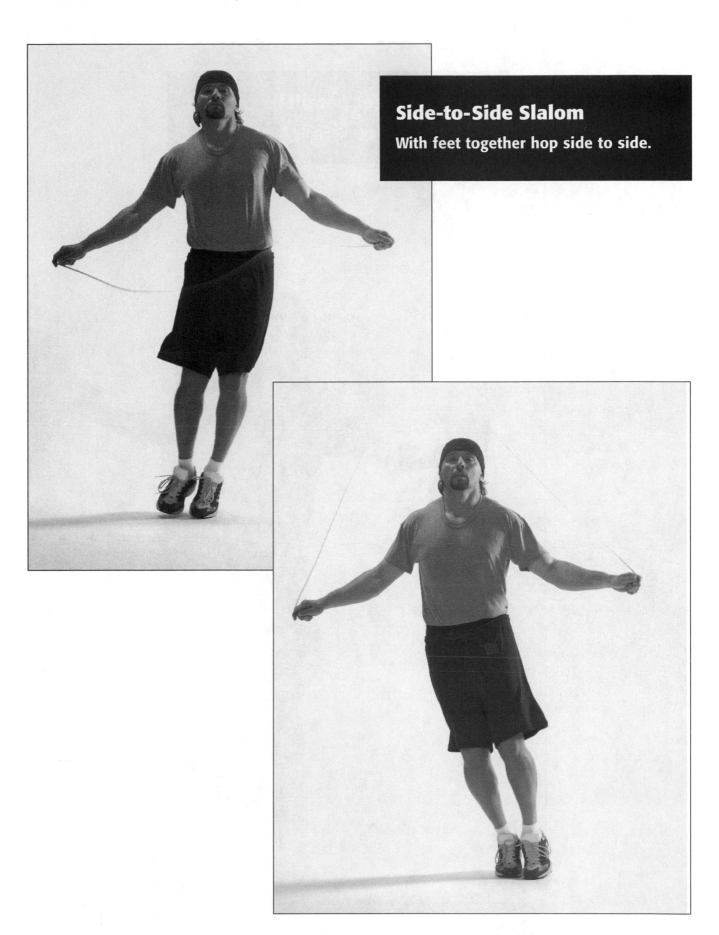

Side-to-Side Slalom
With feet together hop side to side.

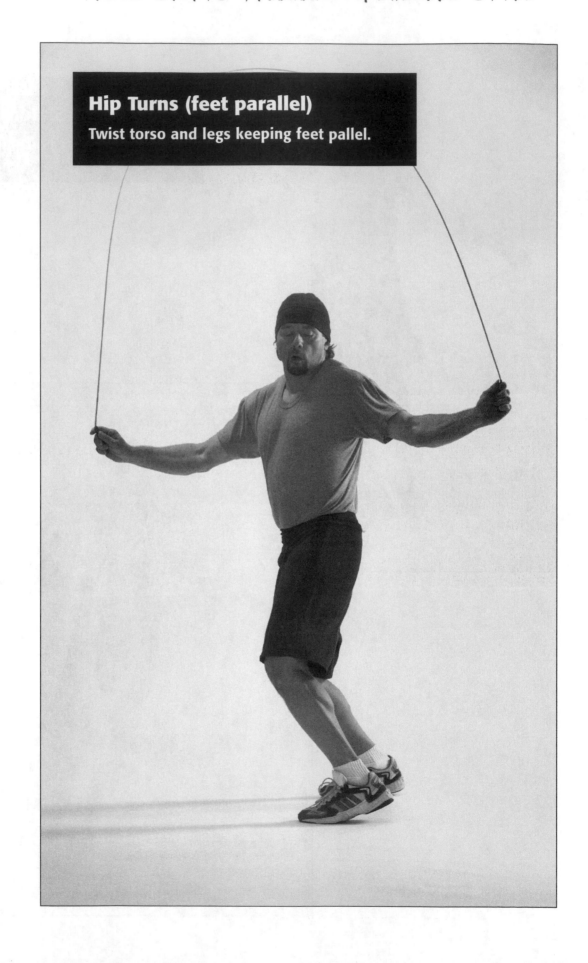

Hip Turns (feet parallel)
Twist torso and legs keeping feet pallel.

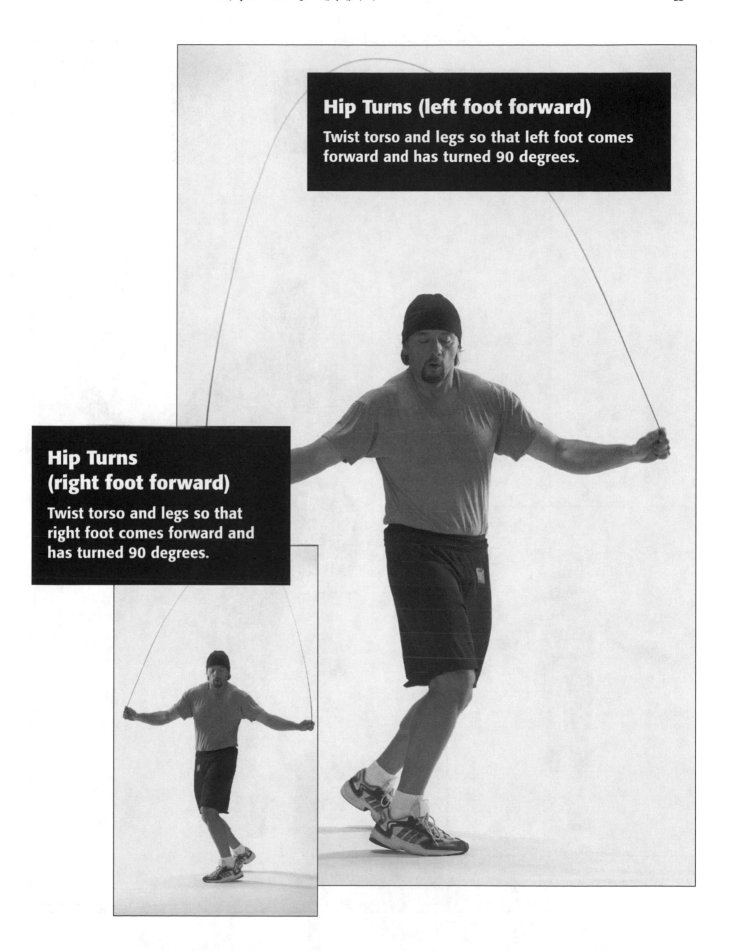

Hip Turns (left foot forward)

Twist torso and legs so that left foot comes forward and has turned 90 degrees.

Hip Turns (right foot forward)

Twist torso and legs so that right foot comes forward and has turned 90 degrees.

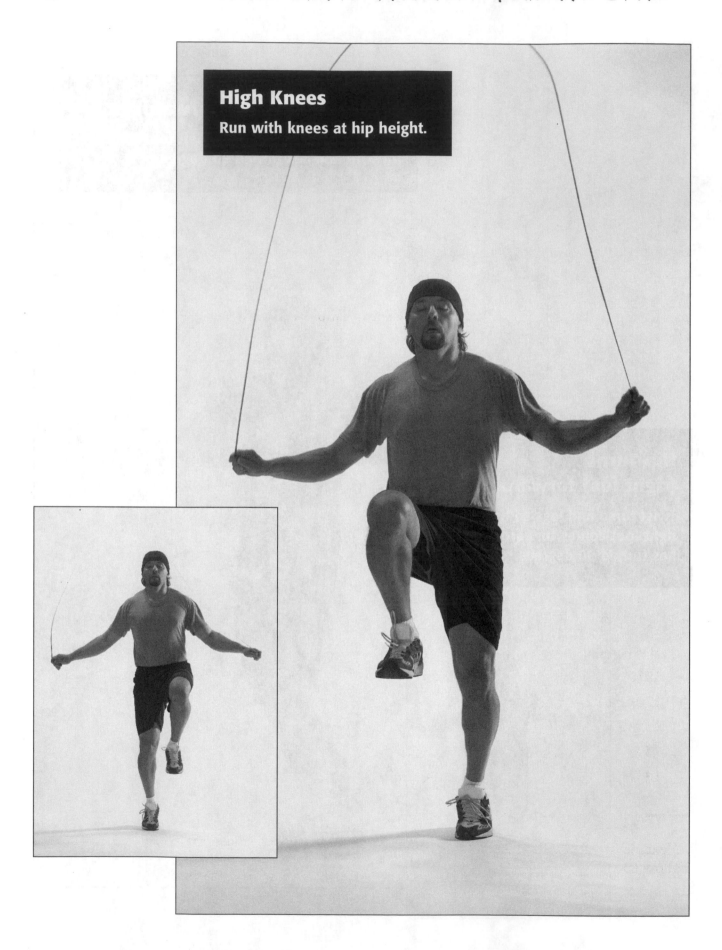

High Knees

Run with knees at hip height.

Without question, when you start skipping rope, you'll find it difficult to complete a full 3-minute round. So you should start with simple 1-minute rounds, and don't vary the movement; also allow 1-minute rest sessions between rounds. Gradually work up to completing 2- and 3-minute rounds, but be patient.

As your work capacity improves, you will perform 3-minute rounds of rope skipping separated by 1-minute active breaks, which comprise a series of exercises. If you maintain a steady regimen of rope work, gradually building up how much you do, you will be astonished at how quickly you advance.

Once you can perform the 3-minute rounds, use the sequence outlined below, in which the movement patterns that I prefer are broken into 15-second splits within the 3-minute rounds. The constant variation of this sequence will provide a physical challenge and a nice degree of variation. You should use the alarm on your watch to signal when to move from one pattern to the next.

Skipping Sequence

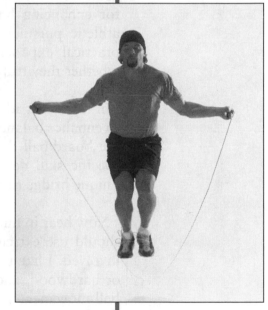

Time	Drill
0–15 seconds	Basic 2 feet together
15–30 seconds	Crossover of hands
30–45 seconds	Ali shuffle
45–60 seconds	Double-skips
60–75 seconds	Side-to-side slalom
75–90 seconds	Crossover of hands
90–105 seconds	Hip turn, feet parallel
105–120 seconds	Crossover of hands
120–135 seconds	Hip turn, left foot forward
135–150 seconds	Crossover of hands
150–165 seconds	Hip turn, right foot forward
165–180 seconds	High knees

Next, let's turn to the exercises done during the 1-minute active breaks. Follow this easy-to-use weekly pattern:

Monday, Wednesday, and Friday

Rounds 1–3: Do fisted pushups for 30 seconds between rounds (but not to the point of failure).

Tuesday and Thursday

Rounds 1–4: Allow complete rest between rounds.

In addition to the various physical benefits of using this type of circuit method, many athletes also notice a heightened sense of awareness or concentration, which they can quickly adapt for their sport of choice. These exercises will coincide with additional work performed in the day.

Balance Training

The Renegade method of balance training is quasi sport-specific training. It uses two mediums—Swiss balls and balance boards—that, as noted earlier, are sometimes considered controversial in the strength and conditioning community. Chiefly, the debate is over the effectiveness of using these mediums for enhancing balance work in traditional sports, like baseball and other athletic pursuits, and the argument is made by individuals who have no practical experience on a board of any kind (which makes me question whether they truly get it).

In my Renegade program, I don't necessarily use, say, the board or the ball to enhance balance in the way most other programs do (although training with the board/ball does enhance balance). Instead, my goal is to enhance sport-specific skill development. And training with the board or ball provides a unique bridge to many of the highly complex, sport-specific maneuvers.

Now bear in mind, these training measures are *extremely advanced,* and you should use extreme caution when starting out, as a bit of falling is usually involved. I like to practice with the board on a fast surface, such as concrete or hardwood, and suggest wearing appropriate pads and helmet. With Swiss ball movements, make sure you have enough space to get off the ball in case you lose your balance, or else have some sort of bracing available to steady yourself.

My point is, *train safely.* You will have to take plenty of chances when you're out there doing your sport!

Balance Board Training

While working on board skills for your sport of choice—be it skateboarding, surfing, wakeboarding, or snowboarding—it's obviously to your advantage to train in your actual sport, with your actual equipment. In fact, nothing can replace your actual time on the board, bike, or blade.

Unfortunately, training under real conditions just isn't always possible, for a variety of reasons. Weather comes to mind, for instance, say, for streetboarders who live in winter climates. Surfers have a similar problem: How can they work on their skills if the waves just aren't there? Or how can their practice their cutback when the waves are inconsistent and the line up is way too cluttered?

Most X-athletes do what they can to accommodate their training. They might ride a stationary bike, for instance. And while some commercial gym settings have balance boards available, most aren't up to the task of doing progressive moves. The bottom line is that training without suitable equipment makes it difficult to work consistently on the same maneuver.

Of the balance boards that are out there, I've found that the *Indo board* meets the needs of athletes of every age and ability. Developed by Hunter Joslin, the Indo line of boards is known primarily within the surfing community, which is unfortunate, because these boards are well-suited to athletes in all the Xtreme sports. In developing the new *Renegade* balance board, I've worked closely with Indo to create the next generation of boards.

The Renegade (manufactured by Indo) is a highly challenging but incredibly responsive board that can be used after working your way through other models of the Indo line. Think of the Renegade as the final board in the progression of boards—the sort of graduate-level deck! It resembles an old-school skate deck but has a larger landing surface and a slightly convex shape that will simulate the heel/toe action demanded by virtually all board sports. The board rests on the same cylinder that the other Indo boards do.

With the Renegade, you can work endlessly on your skills, developing foot/board awareness and trunk stability and practicing the most complex of tricks. Or you can use the board to perform simple balancing maneuvers, which are important whether you are a board sport athlete, a trail rider, or a "flatlander."

Critics will comment that by practicing an exercise on a balance board, you will learn to perform that exercise *only* on that board and be unable to transfer what you've learned to the actual sport. This isn't true for board sport athletes. You will be able to transfer what you've learned because, in fact, you *will* work on your balance in an environment that's very similar to that of many Xtreme sports. And given this carryover, it will be extremely useful to anyone who wants to learn tricks and maneuvers on a board or who wants to improve balance on a BMX or MTB bike (not to mention rehabilitate from injuries).

Let me emphasize just how important balance is to Xtreme sports. Unless you achieve the total body awareness that comes with balance training, your performance skills as an X-athlete will be limited. In saying this, I don't mean to de-emphasize the importance of the other elements of the wheel of conditioning (first mentioned in Chapter 1), such as agility training and range of motion development. All of these elements should be developed equally. But without complete balance and control, your ultimate performance will suffer—and you'll know it!

All athletes, not just board sport athletes, should work on the exercises listed below, as doing so will enhance a variety of skills, such as balance, torso speed, and stability. Skateboarders, in particular, will be able to perform these movements with ease, but doing them will benefit everyone. Take your time and be patient. You should perform the following drills daily on the balance board without exception:

- Squats
- Ollies
- Shuv-its
- Cut-backs

And if you're a surfer, you should do these daily drills, as well:

- Pop-ups
- Hang 10s
- Boardwalks
- Pipeline stances

The specific amount of time you should spend on the board is broken out in the training program supplied in Chapter 7 on Specialized Physical Preparation (SPP). You can certainly spend *additional* time on the board, however, and may well want to because it rocks! Just keep in mind that these are highly advanced exercises. Don't expect them to be easy.

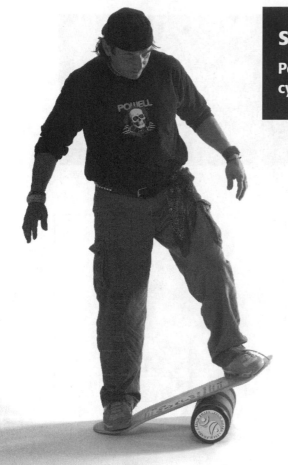

Squats

Position board at top 1/3 resting on cyclinder, relax at knees.

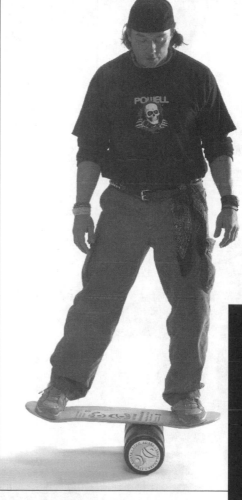

Shoot board forward as you drop-in with just enough speed but ease back and center board ~ relax.

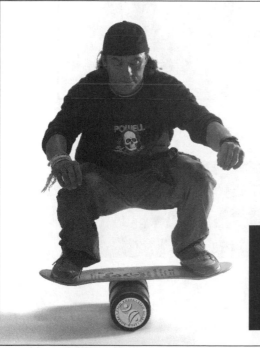

Simultaneously push butt back and bend at knees while you squat down.

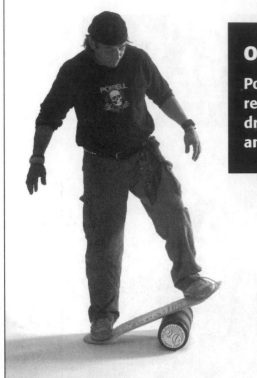

Ollies

Position board at top 1/3 resting on cyclinder, relax at knees, shoot board forward as you drop-in with just enough speed but ease back and center board ~ relax.

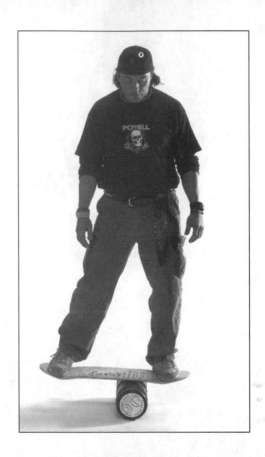

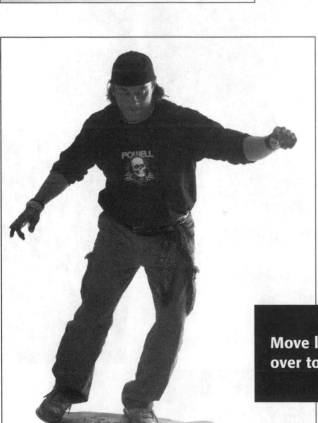

Move lead foot back such that it is over top of cylinder.

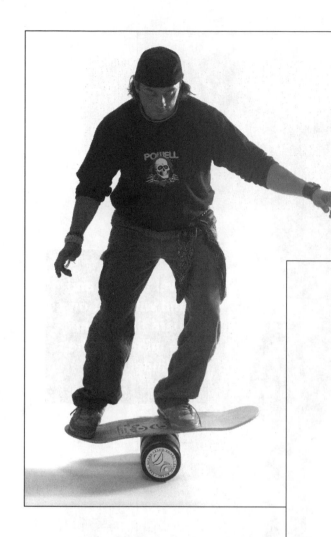

Snap back foot down while simultaneously dragging lead foot up, in fact drawing board upwards.

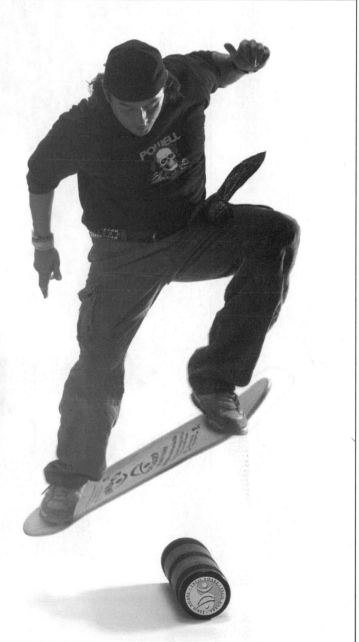

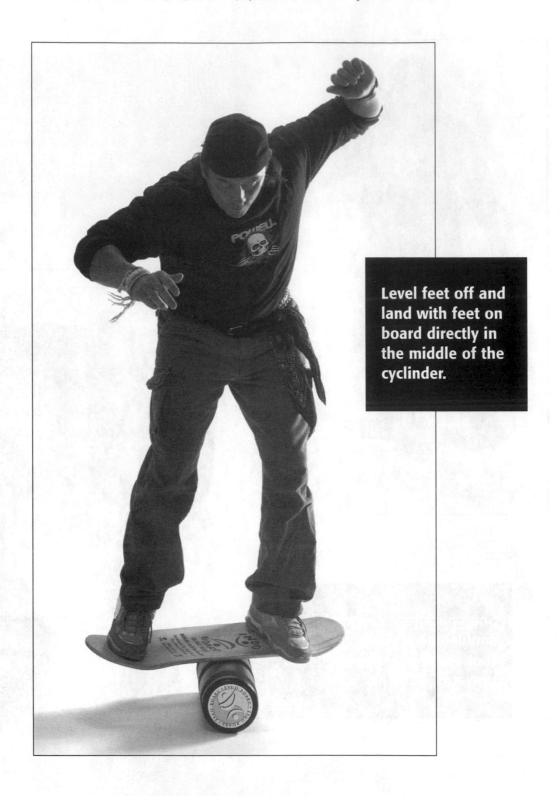

Level feet off and land with feet on board directly in the middle of the cyclinder.

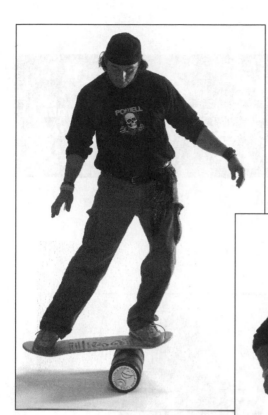

Shuv-its

In fact – a balance board style Shuv-it for the purists but after centering up on board, pull board again such that front foot is near cyclinder.

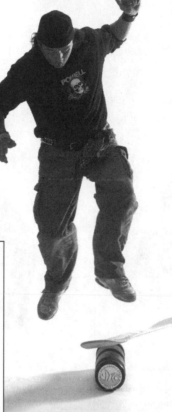

Shoot board back twisting board behind you rotating board on cyclinder as you jump up drawing knees up.

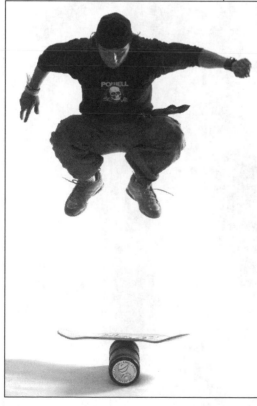

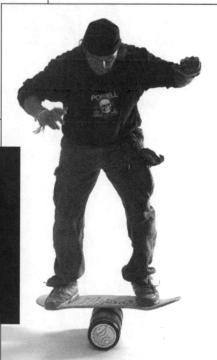

land both feet on board simultaneiously with the board directly in the middle of the cyclinder.

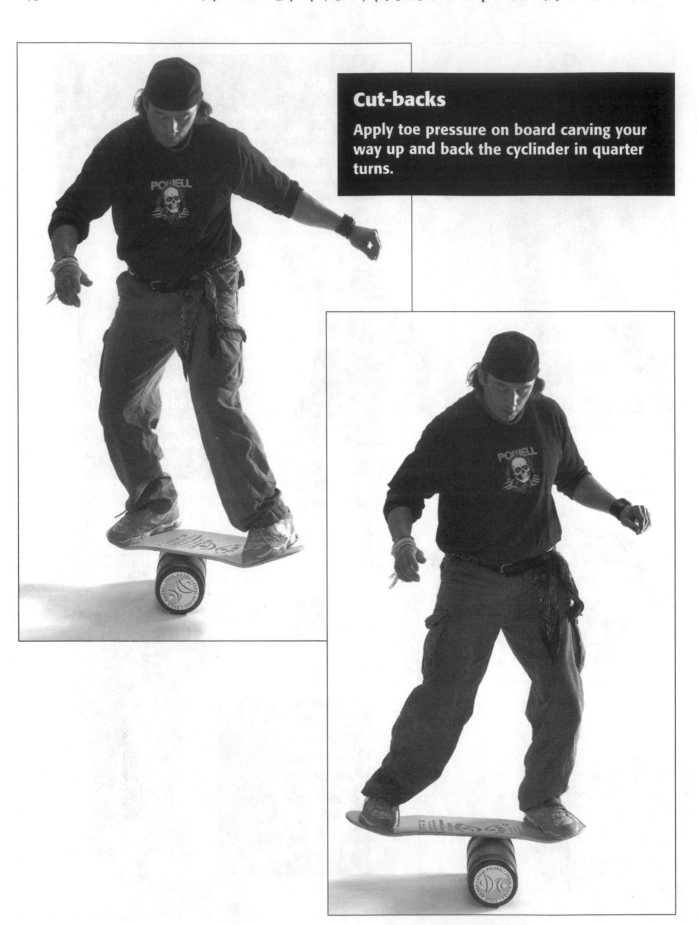

Cut-backs

Apply toe pressure on board carving your way up and back the cyclinder in quarter turns.

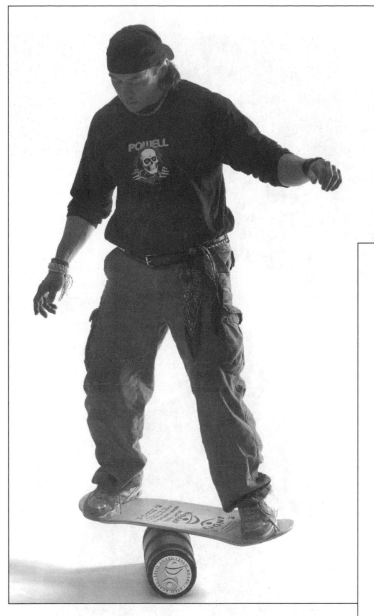

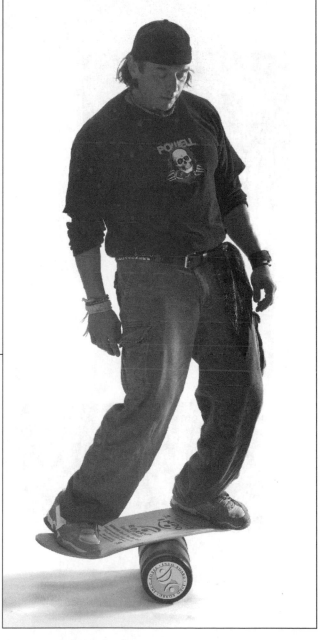

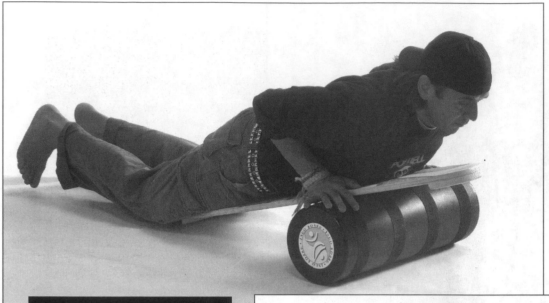

Pop-ups

Using the Surf Pro model – laying on the ground with top 1/3 of board over cyclinder.

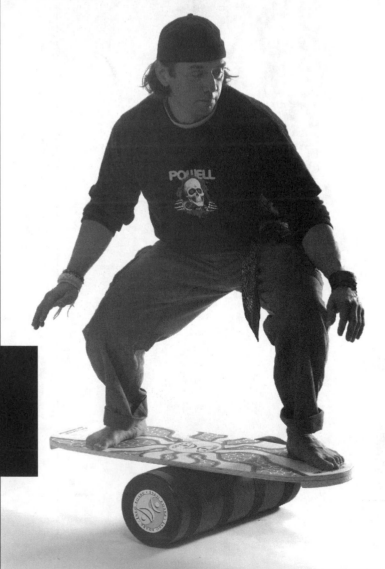

Shoot board with extraordinary speed, compressing immediately into pipeline stance.

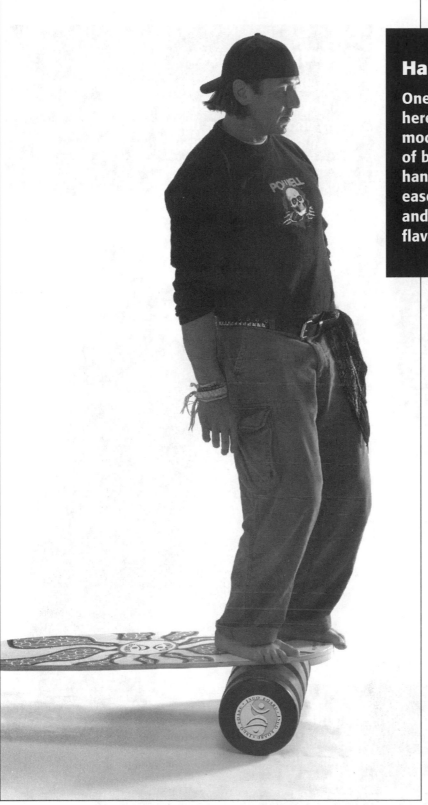

Hang 10s

One for the style council here, using the Surf Pro model – walk to the front of board until toes are hanging over edge and ease hips waaaay forward and lean back – add some flavor.

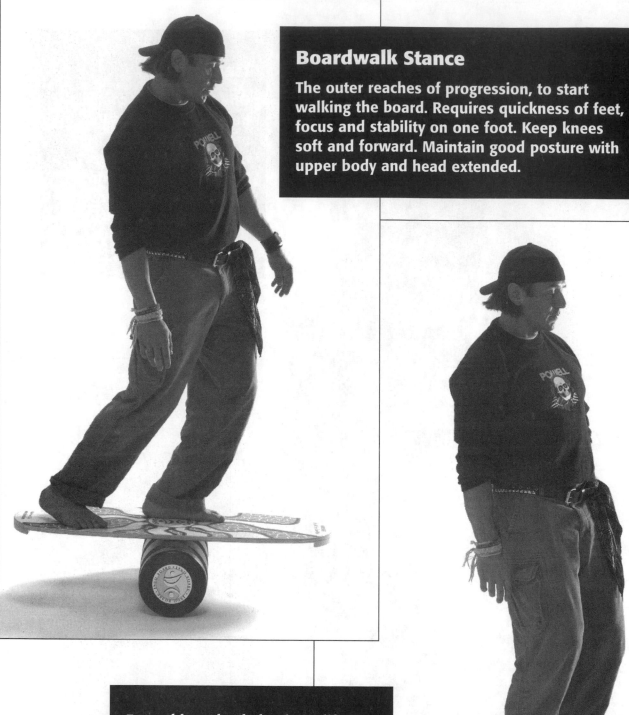

Boardwalk Stance

The outer reaches of progression, to start walking the board. Requires quickness of feet, focus and stability on one foot. Keep knees soft and forward. Maintain good posture with upper body and head extended.

From this – slowly begin to lift one foot and bring one foot behind the other. Be patient this will take time but pay off big.

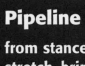

Pipeline

from stance position execute pipeline as in stretch, bringing back knee/shin to board keeping lead hand by knee and back hand pressing against that wall.

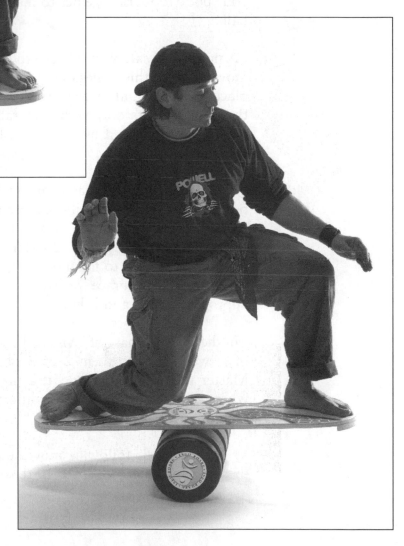

Swiss Ball Training

Some will argue that Swiss balls are intended more for orthopedic use than for athletic development. However, this medium has drawn considerable attention within the fitness community after being introduced by practitioners such as the well-published Paul Chek. Swiss ball advocates note that this is an effective medium for enhancing stabilization strength, for re-educating the neuromuscular system, and for improving general balance and control.

Some members of the scientific community will debate the effectiveness of working with Swiss balls in comparison with, say, performing certain Olympic lifts. From my view, this debate is irrelevant because the Renegade program uses Swiss balls to enhance the sport-specific skills of Xtreme sports. When you think about learning to control the board or keeping your balance over rough terrain while doing jumps and so forth, it becomes clear that the unstable surface of the ball provides an appropriate (albeit imperfect) setting for training. The ball offers a unique resistance, forcing the various parts of your body to work together to maintain balance and control the edges of the ball.

A number of safety issues need to be considered with Swiss ball training. The movements in this Renegade program, in particular, are highly advanced and place great demand on the structure of the ball. I strongly recommend doing these movements only with a Duraball, which is nonburstable up to 1,000 pounds of pressure if used and cared for properly. An inferior ball will likely burst and cause injury.

Another safety issue has to do with the setting in which you train. When performing any of the drills, choose a place in which you have enough room to maneuver. You need to be able to get off the ball in case you start to lose your balance, and if you do start to go down, you don't want to have equipment around to fall into. You may, however, want to use a wall against which you can brace or steady yourself. Finally, be sure to wear the appropriate pads and helmet.

In the earliest phase of Swiss ball work, I start with the following progression of movements. Do them 2 or 3 times a week by training every other day. Master the movements one at a time, adding a new one in each session or whenever you are completely comfortable in doing so. You should gauge your own progress.

For each of the following movements, hold the position for 15 seconds and then rest for 45 seconds. Do 10 reps per set and 3 to 5 sets.

Beginning Swiss Ball Movements

- Sit on the ball, your back straight and your hands on your thighs.
- Sit on the ball, your back straight and your arms stretched out in front of you, parallel to the ground.
- Sit on the ball, your back straight and your arms stretched straight overhead.
- Sit on your haunches on the ball, your hands on your thighs.
- Sit on your haunches on the ball, your arms stretched out in front of you, parallel to ground.
- Kneel on the ball, your hands on your thighs.
- Kneel on the ball, your arms stretched out in front of you, parallel to ground.

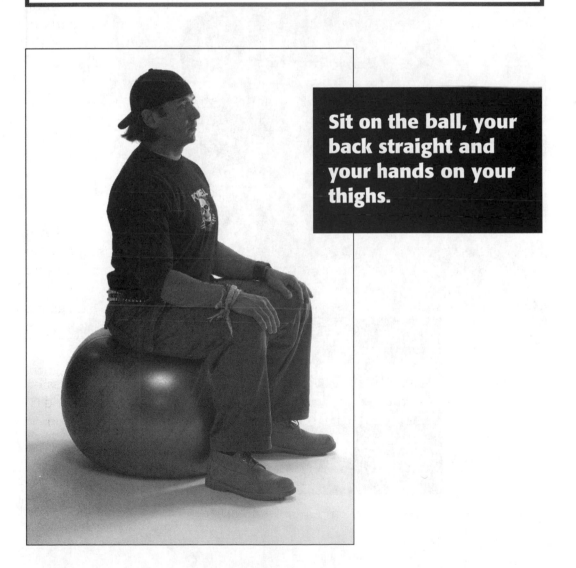

Sit on the ball, your back straight and your hands on your thighs.

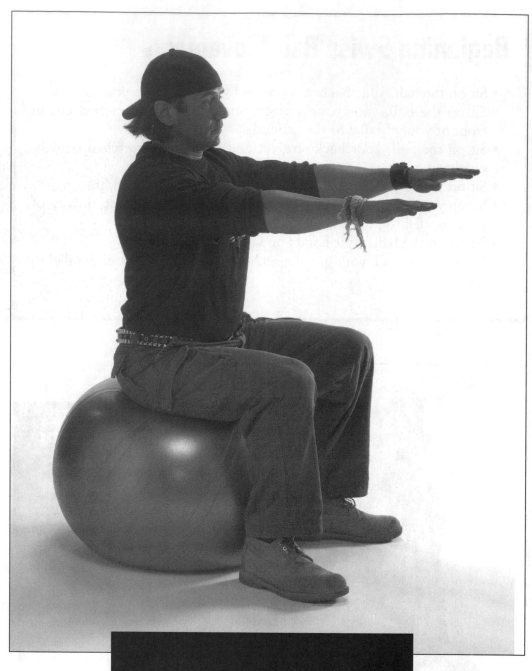

Sit on the ball, your back straight and your arms stretched out in front of you, parallel to the ground.

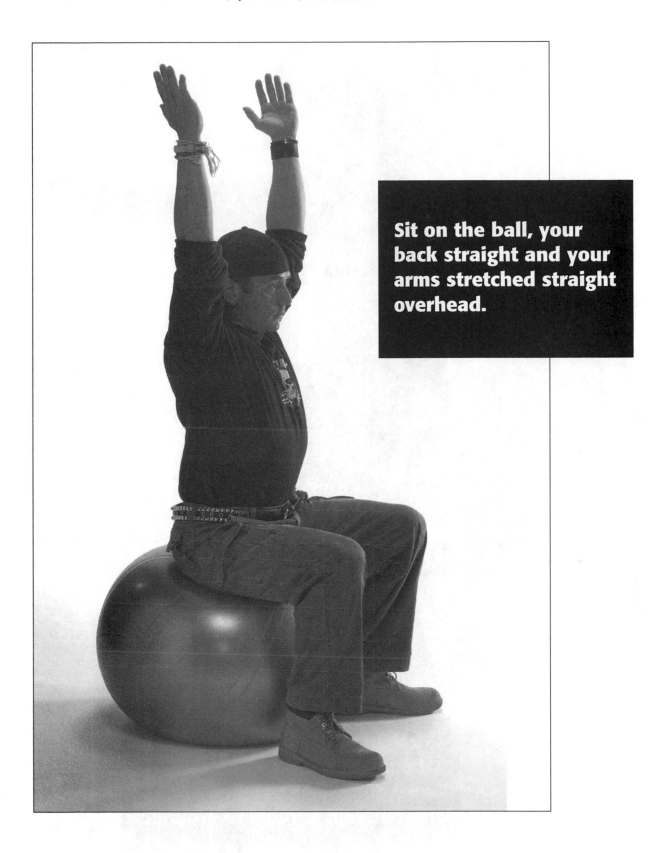

Sit on the ball, your back straight and your arms stretched straight overhead.

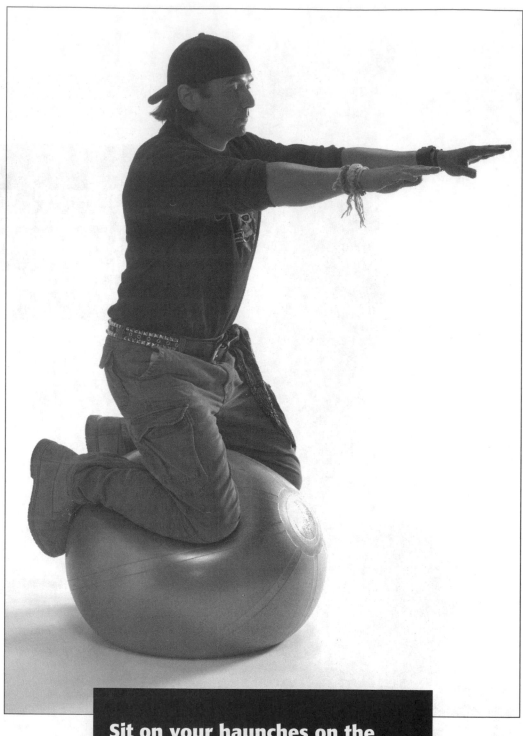

Sit on your haunches on the ball, your arms stretched out in front of you, parallel to ground.

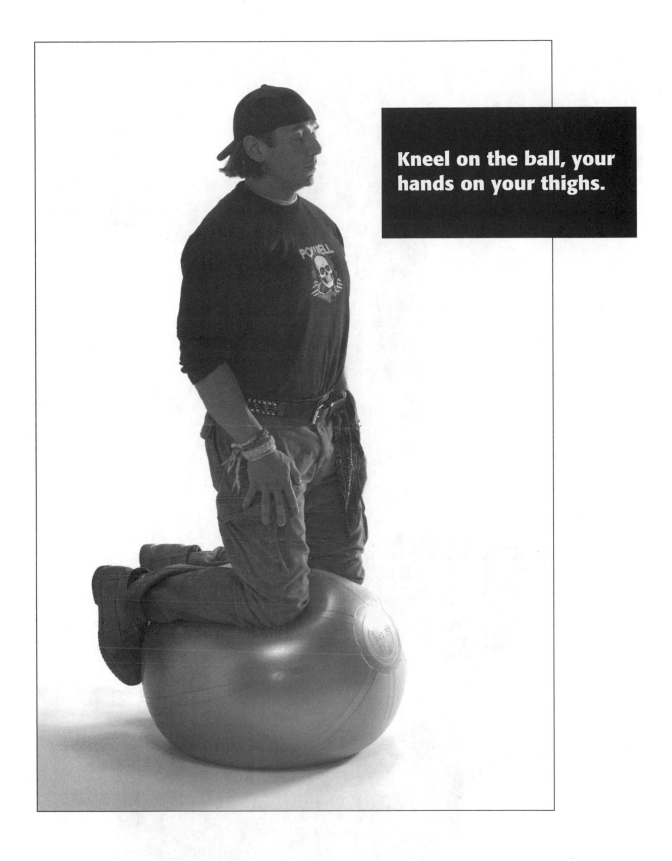

Kneel on the ball, your hands on your thighs.

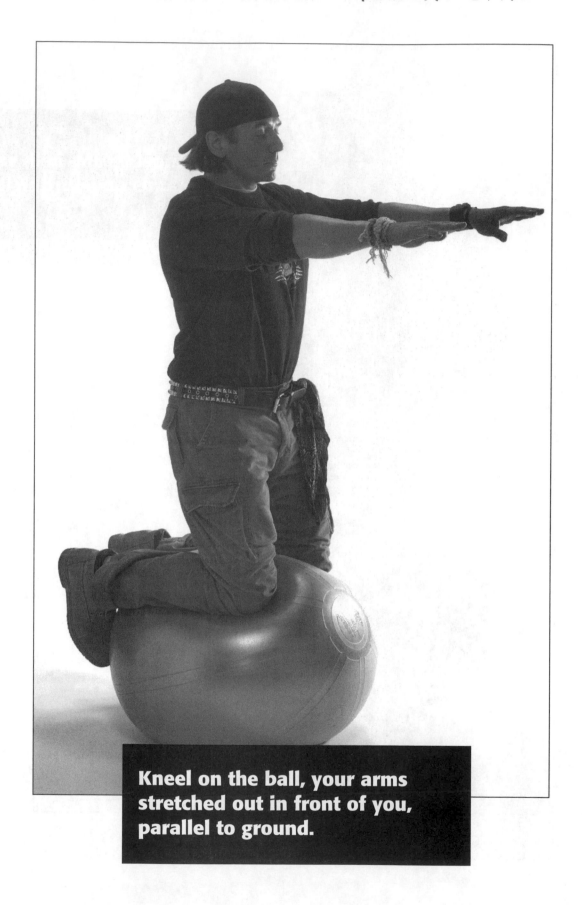

Kneel on the ball, your arms stretched out in front of you, parallel to ground.

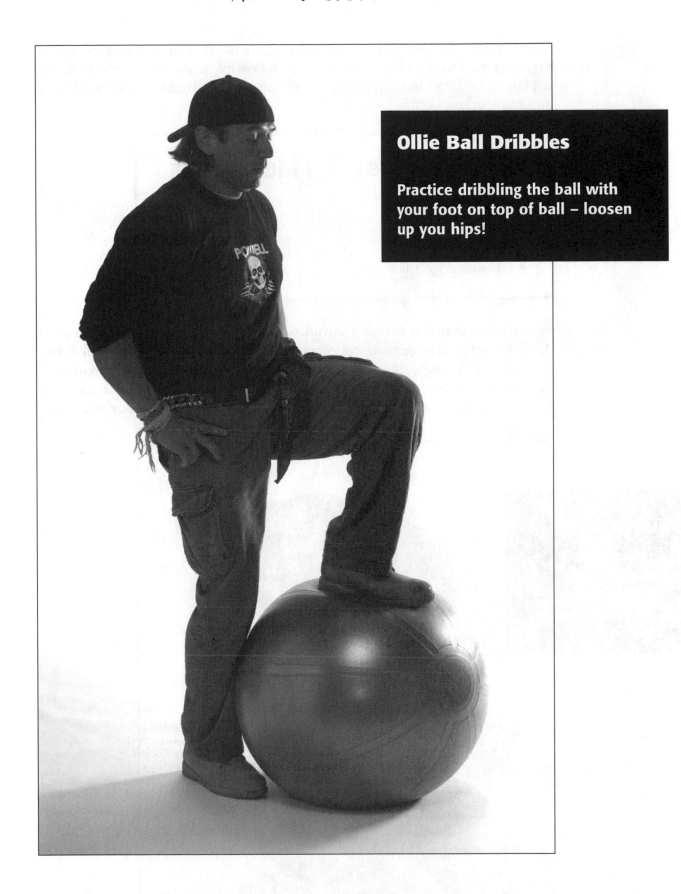

Ollie Ball Dribbles

Practice dribbling the ball with your foot on top of ball – loosen up you hips!

Once you've mastered these beginning movements, you can progress to the mainstay of Swiss ball training. Do the following drills on a daily basis (as explained in detail in Chapter 7) in order to develop tremendous board sense and tremendous control.

Advanced Swiss Ball Movements

- Ollie ball dribbles
- Squats
- Back-and-forth rolls
- Outside-edge rolls

Remember that this is highly advanced work, and you shouldn't attempt to do it without taking the proper precautions. Be extremely careful when starting out! To reiterate, use a safe ball and wear the appropriate pads and helmet. Also make sure you have enough space to get off the ball in case you lose your balance, or have some sort of bracing available to steady yourself.

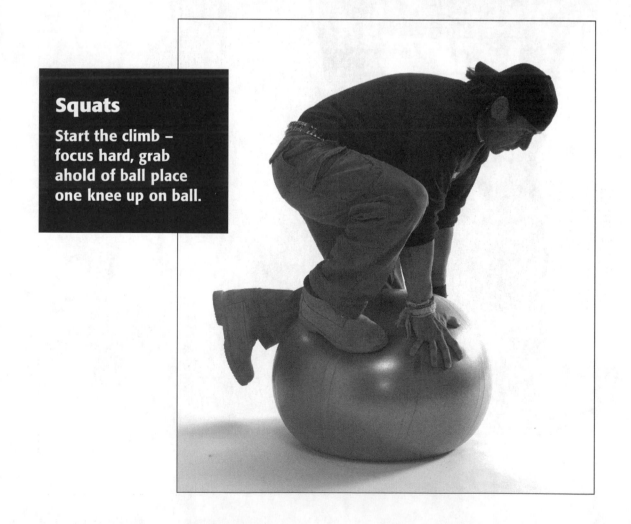

Squats

Start the climb – focus hard, grab ahold of ball place one knee up on ball.

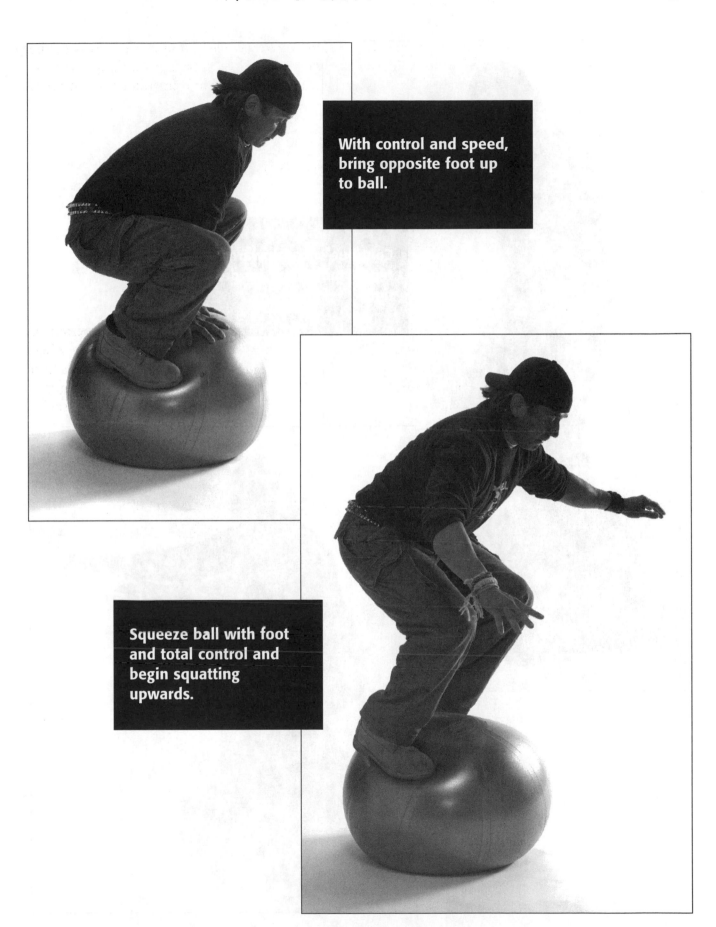

With control and speed, bring opposite foot up to ball.

Squeeze ball with foot and total control and begin squatting upwards.

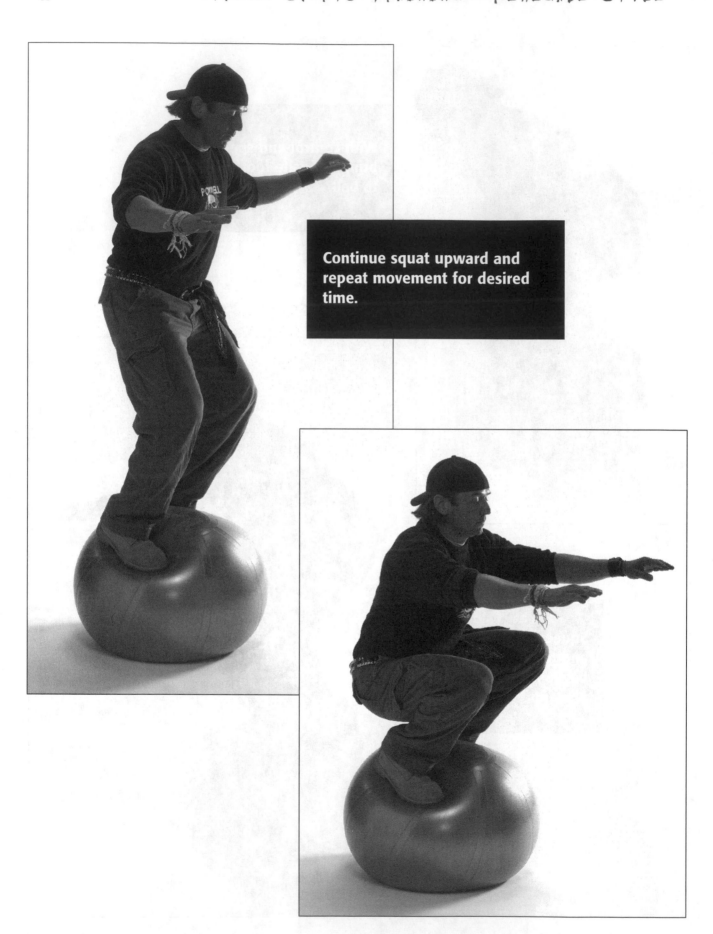

Continue squat upward and repeat movement for desired time.

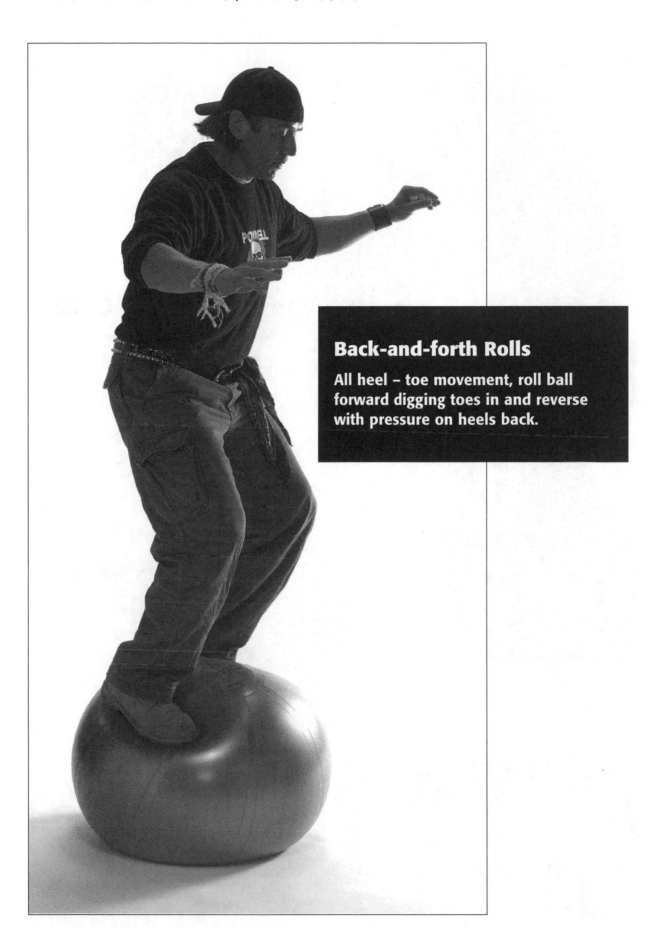

Back-and-forth Rolls

All heel – toe movement, roll ball forward digging toes in and reverse with pressure on heels back.

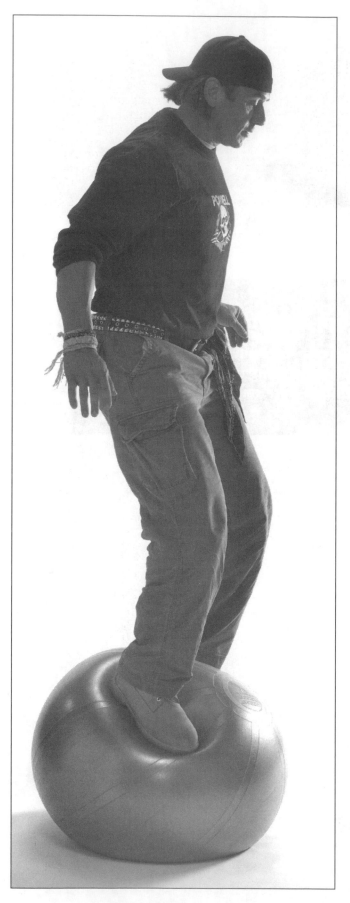
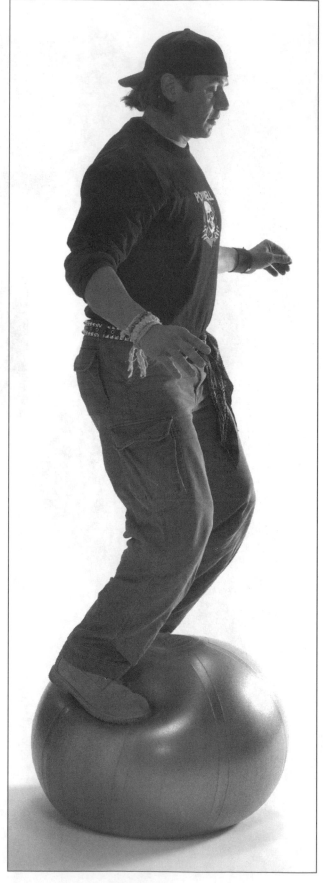

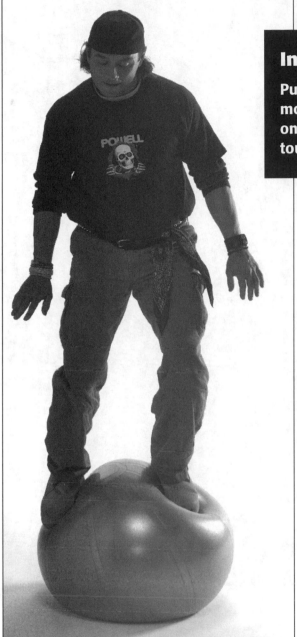

Inside/Outside-Edge Rolls

Pull ball by loosening hold with one foot and moving ball to opposite side until one foot is on side of ball. Be patient with this – this is a tough test of strength and control.

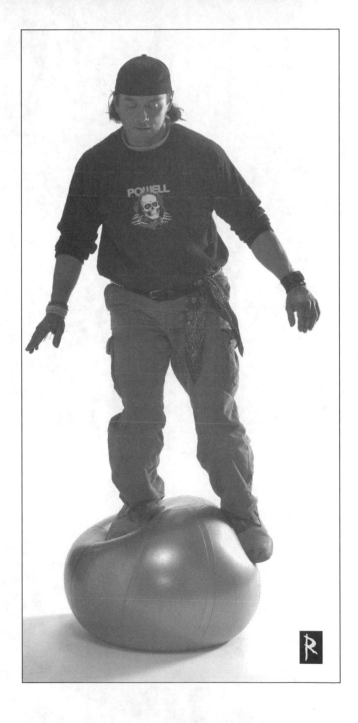

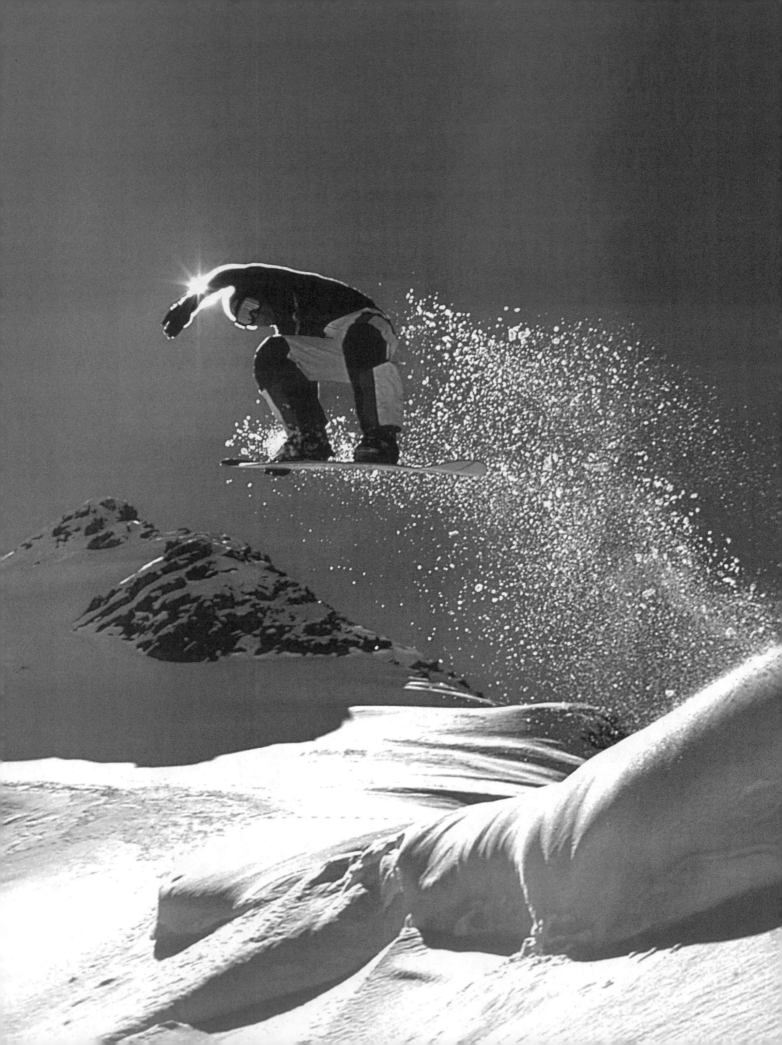

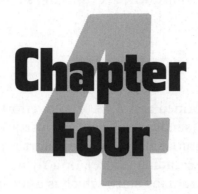

Chapter Four

How to Gain Awesome Speed and Xplosive Jumping Power

In the realm of Xtreme sports, speed and explosive jump training is more focused on sport-specific performance on the board or the bike, not necessarily on sprint form and technique. In fact, spending endless time on perfecting sprinting form is not warranted or worthwhile for the X-athlete, and training in this area is somewhat less complicated than in other areas.

Improving absolute speed and cxplosive power is, in fact, a by-product of the work that you've done in the balance of the Renegade Training program. And the purpose of improving speed and power in the Xtreme sports is to attain optimal speed in your sessions and maximum height in your jumps, ollies, and so forth. Toward those goals, the Renegade "plan of attack" uses several sprint patterns and a plyometric jump training drill.

Sprint Patterns

To offer variation in training and to maximize improvement in linear speed, sprint work is broken into maximal work and submaximal work. As explained below, these are essentially difficulty levels and should be completed at different time intervals. Having these two types of sprint work allows you to combine different levels in your weekly training—say, Sequence A from the maximal work group with Sequence A from the submaximal group.

Maximal Work Sequences

Maximal work is performed at 100% of total effort, and sessions should be at least 72 hours apart. As indicated below, each sequence begins from a laying (supine) position start (initiated by a "clap" start signal), a 2-point standing start (which is a regular, standing stance), or a flying 10-yard start. (Note that a flying start is simply a running start, which is done by gradually accelerating to the start line with a 10-yard lead-in.) In addition to the position start, the yardage and repeats (or number of times to perform) are provided for each sprint.

Sequence A

75 yards x 2, from flying 10-yard start
50 yards x 2, from supine "clap" start
65 yards x 2, from 2-point standing start
20 yards x 2, from supine "clap" start

Sequence B

55 yards x 2, from flying 10-yard start
25 yards x 3, from supine "clap" start
40 yards x 2, from 2-point standing start
10 yards x 3, from supine "clap" start

Submaximal Work Sequences

Submaximal work is performed at 70% of total effort, and sessions should be at least 24 to 48 hours apart. The emphasis is on proper form. These sprint sequences are sometimes called *tempo runs* or *circuit runs*.

Sequence A

100 x 3, with 20-yard walk between intervals, rest 90 seconds
100, 100 x 2, 100, with 20-yard walk between intervals, rest 90 seconds
100 x 2, 100, 100 x 2, with 20-yard walk between intervals, rest 90 seconds
100, 100 x 2, 100, with 20-yard walk between intervals, rest 90 seconds
100 x 3, with 20-yard walk between intervals

Sequence B

75 yards x 3 repeats, with 20-yard walk between intervals, rest 90 seconds

75 yards, 75 yards x 2 (back and forth), 75 yards, with 20-yard walk between intervals, rest 90 seconds

75 yards x 2 repeats, 75 yards, 75 x 2 (back and forth), with 20-yard walk between intervals, rest 90 seconds

75 yards, 75 yards x 2, 75 yards, with 20-yard walk between intervals, rest 90 seconds

75 yards x 3 repeats, with 20-yard walk between intervals

Plyometric Training

Plyometric training was first used in the United States after "emigrating" with European coaches and being dubbed the "secret training protocol" of the Soviet Union. Work on these *shock drills,* as they are sometimes called, was pioneered through the extraordinary effort of Soviet coach Yuri V. Verkhoshansky.

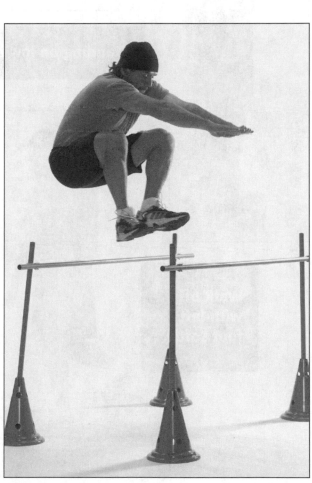

Technically speaking, plyometric drills are performed to develop an eccentric muscle contraction followed by a concentric muscle contraction, which is known as a *stretch-shortening cycle.* The idea is to condition the muscles to making sudden moves in opposite directions, ultimately generating greater force and power. The application of plyometrics to many of the Xtreme sports is obvious, as having explosive power and being able to "get air" is paramount to success. Thus, training in this area is of extraordinary importance, and its value cannot be underestimated.

Nonetheless, it's imperative that plyometric work be done only after significant muscular conditioning has been achieved. Make sure you start from a solid foundation. The Renegade approach builds on this foundation in a controlled manner, such that you can maximize your results. While many different drills (and mediums) can be used, I have found that three offer tremendous results in enhancing the movements of the lower extremities:

Box Triple Jump

One of the best jump drills for developing explosive power is the box triple jump. All athletes will benefit from the increased explosive power that comes from doing this jump, but skateboarders, especially, will see that the height of the lift knee in this move is similar to that in lifting the board when ollie-ing. To perform this jump, start by standing on a short box—one that's approximately 1 foot high. Walk off the box slowly, leading with your left leg and landing it flat. Follow with a quick impulse jump forward with the right leg, driving your knee up as high as possible. The total distance of the jump should be approximately 2 feet between each foot. As your right foot contacts the ground, drive your left knee up and as high as possible. Continue with a repeat jump of the right leg and so on.

Standing on low box.

Walk off with left foot softly.

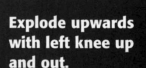

Explode upwards with left knee up and out.

High box jump (not pictured)

Start by standing in front of a box that's 36 to 42 inches high. In an explosive movement, jump up and on top of the box. Upon contact, immediately jump off and out as high and as far as possible. Land in a low tuck position. For safety, be sure to wear proper shoes and land on a stable surface at all times.

Barrier Jump

Place five hurdles, with the barrier set at hip height, roughly 3 feet apart. Standing in front of the first hurdle, relax and leap over it. As you land, quickly explode and leap over the next hurdle. Continue in this manner until you've cleared all five hurdles. Repeat as directed in the training program provided in Chapter 7. Perform this exercise with an element of "flow." Allow your body to learn how to perform a difficult maneuver in an easy manner.

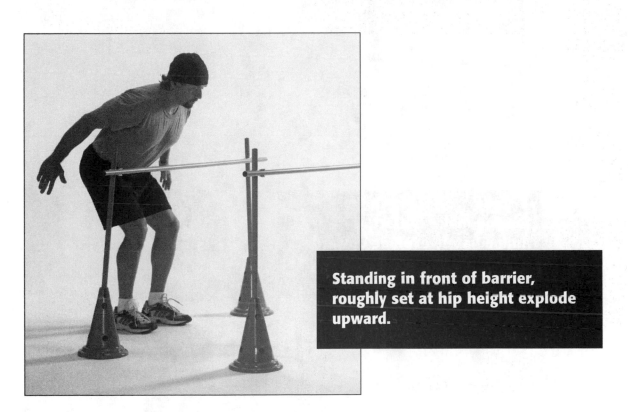

Standing in front of barrier, roughly set at hip height explode upward.

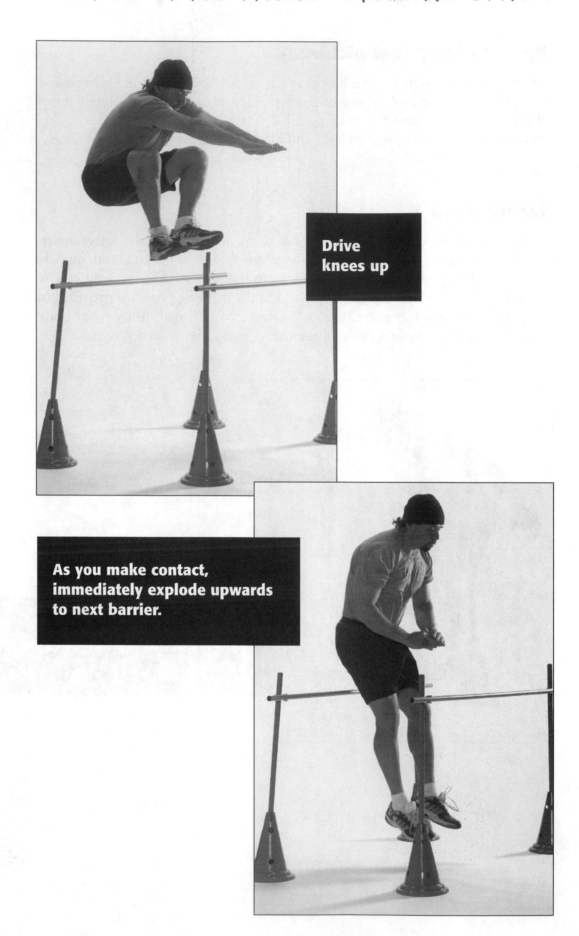

Drive knees up

As you make contact, immediately explode upwards to next barrier.

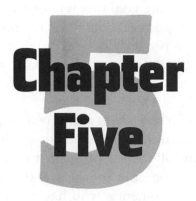

Chapter Five

Xtreme Toughness— Developing The Strength You Need to Master Mean Curves, Hellacious Waves, and Brutal Tracks

As with other areas of the Renegade approach, training in strength development is based entirely on improving performance in your sport of choice. In the simplest terms, nothing is done if it doesn't enhance performance, whether that means getting more air, being able to paddle out in tougher surf, or being resistant to those ever-daunting injuries.

Yet strength training in the Xtreme arena is particularly complex and, in fact, extraordinarily new. Given this, many X-athletes aren't accustomed to strength training. For years, much of the information available to them seemed to focus on just getting buff and was prepared by someone who had no insight into their sport.

This isn't the case with the Renegade "plan of attack," which is rooted in a careful understanding of what it takes to succeed in these sports. Strength work is done for a reason you may never have considered or even heard of.

It's not to look buff or to put on unnecessary muscle. (Neither will make you ride better.) Rather the ultimate goal of strength training is to possess a total body awareness and better postural alignment to enhance sport performance. Toward that goal, having a properly designed strength program will give you give you such things as greater pop on your board and the ability to charge through the toughest of runs. Again, improving performance is the key.

Another benefit of strength training is that it will help you develop the ability to resist injury from those nasty spills and tosses that are basic to X-treme sports. Getting hurt is an all-to-real problem for the X-athlete. Even so, a stronger, fitter athlete will be able to withstand the punishment of, say, a pounding wave better than someone who has not trained in this area. And believe me, I can speak from experience here, as I've bitten it pretty bad on more than one occasion! If you stay fit, strong, and pliable, you will be more resistant to getting hurt. It's that simple!

One basic element of the Renegade approach is to use a wide variety of exercise movements, which has several benefits. First of all, consistently varying exercise stimuli helps avoid muscular adaptation, in which the body adapts to training and results lag in a sort of "law of diminishing returns." This is a key long-term principle in many training programs. In addition, varying exercise movements creates a training consequence of improved motor skill ability, which will synergistically translate into sport-specific skills, whether you're on a board or a bike.

The Renegade "plan of attack" is also known for being relentless and creating an element of chaos that proves invaluable in training for Xtreme sports. Those of you who are accustomed to feeling the adrenaline rush that comes from doing these sports will know what I'm talking about here. You will feel the same sort of rush in training the Renegade way as you do during a great session on your board or bike. We Renegades train as we ride: full out, with no holding back.

The Basics of Lifting

Underlying the Renegade approach to lifting is the understanding that the body has three planes of motion:

1. The *coronal plane* cuts the front and back portions of the body.
2. The *sagittal plane* cuts the right and the left segments of the body.
3. The *transverse plane* divides the top and the bottom parts of the body.

With this as its foundation, the Renegade strength program uses nonweighted movements, multiple-joint lifts, and lifting complexes, each done in a fashion to teach the individual parts of the body to work in a harmonious fashion. The simple cornerstones of the program are pushing, pulling, rotating, lungeing, and squatting motions. And several mediums are used—typically, either barbells or kettlebells.

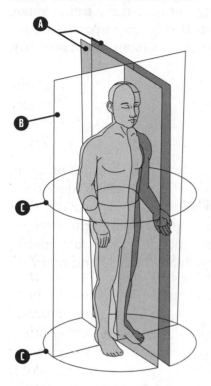

Body Planes

A. The Sagittal plane, also called the Median plane can be broken into Perimedian planes anywhere across the body. Anatomy is defined by left and right or lateral and medial relations in this plane.

B. The Coronal plane or frontal plane falls on the Coronal suture of the skull. Anatomy is defined by Anterior and Posterior or Ventral and Dorsal relations in this plane.

C. The Transverse plane, or horizontal plane can fall anywhere on the body, a common midpoint is the navel. Anatomy is defined by cranial and caudal or proximal and distal relations in this plane.

Barbells

The Renegade lifting regime uses only simple weights, no machines, for a very specific reason. While machines can be quite effective in many training environments, they limit range of motion, isolate musculature, and reduce the role of the body's stabilizing muscles (for instance, when performing a standing lift). These are significant limitations if you consider the extraordinary command of balance and control required to perform Xtreme sports. Thus, with few exceptions, the use of machines for strength training is strictly non-Renegade.

The entire strength component of this program can be performed with a simple set of barbells. There's no need to be extravagant and get a fancy, expensive set, which is a particular plus for first-time lifters and anyone who trains at home. Through the use of barbells (and kettlebells, discussed below), you will heighten your body's awareness of and ultimately improve its balance.

Granted, you won't be able to load the same weight on a barbell as you can on a machine, but that's inconsequential for your goal here. In fact, the Renegade approach avoids using heavy weights, recognizing that it's not the weight itself but the speed and control with which you move it that's important. Let me emphasize that *speed and control* go together. You don't want to throw or jerk the weight.

Yet another unique aspect of this program is that you will perform one-armed lifts that many lifters would typically perform using dumbbells. Using barbells makes these lifts particularly taxing, as it places greater demands on the muscles that provide balance and stabilizing—and in the Xtreme game, that's paramount to success. So, whether your goal is to pop up or cut back faster, to charge into a run with more speed or to get more air, done properly, this "plan of attack" will get you there.

Kettlebells

Kettlebell work is an instrumental portion of the Renegade strength program because it's tremendously effective. Athletes who lift kettlebells develop a superb understanding of muscular harmony in addition to improving their balance and developing powerful tendons suitable for long-term strength work. Like barbells, kettlebells offer a training medium that's affordable, especially considering that their period of use is virtually endless and that they are fully transportable.

Types of Lifts

In the chart that follows, you'll see that there are three categories of lifts:

- Focus lifts
- Hybrid lifts
- Supplemental lifts

There are several different movements within each of these three categories, and specific descriptions and illustrations are provided for all of them later in this chapter. But for now, here is a basic explanation of each category of lift.

Focus Lifts

As their name implies, focus lifts are the basic exercises on which this training program is built. Doing these generally multiple-joint, compound movements will reinforce the need for the body's various parts to work in a single, harmonious fashion.

In performing the focus lifts, your work intensity should be in the 40% to 65% range of maximal effort. Perform 6 repetitions (reps) and 3 to 5 sets of each lift, such that the total rep count varies from 18 to 30 during each weight workout. Once you become more technically proficient and confident at these lifts, you will see how they evolve into the training complexes mentioned later. For now, be sure to use a training load that falls within the guidelines, and control the weight with perfect flow and balance.

Hybrid Lifts

This program doesn't use the classic competitive Olympic lifts. Instead, it uses hybrids of those lifts because while the classic lifts are effective for training many athletes (most notably, weightlifters), X-athletes don't need to master the lifts to the same technical degree. In fact, by using the hybrid lifts and unilateral counterparts, you will not only derive the same benefits of enhanced power, speed, and body harmony, but you will also see greater gains in the areas of balance and control.

As outlined in the training program in Chapter 7, these lifts are to be completed in a manner that will maximize explosive and reactive strength without causing unnecessary muscular growth. This is a very important concept, as starting strength, reactive strength, and acceleration strength must be maximized to ensure maximum sport production. To quote Dr. Mel C. Siff, in *Supertraining 2000*, "Starting strength is the ability to quickly develop the greatest possible force at the initial moment of tension" and "Acceleration strength is the ability to build up working force as rapidly as possible once contraction has occurred."

Thus, Renegade strength training is done with maximum bar speed, generating a dynamic force. When doing the hybrid lifts, your work intensity should be 40% to 65% of maximal effort. Again, for each lift, do 6 reps and 3 to 5 sets.

Supplemental Lifts

The supplemental lifts are technically the least challenging of all the lifts, but they are important, nonetheless. Because you are not focusing on the technical difficulty of the lifts, you can focus on how harmoniously your body is working, thus enhancing balance and control. This is especially beneficial for those just who are lifting weights for the first time. doing these supplemental lifts will also help stabilize often injured areas, such as the shoulder capsule and knee.

Complex Lifts

Before moving on, let me also introduce a more advanced type of lift that will be explained in more detail later in the chapter. In the *complex lifts*, the focus lifts have been compounded in order to increase power production, improve endurance, and teach the parts of the body to work harmony. Like the other types of lifts, the complex lifts can be performed with either a barbells or kettlebells. Doing these lifts will have tremendous benefits for your total physiological system.

You'll see that these complexes are slowly written into the training program in Chapter 7, and they provide some of the best and most important elements of Renegade strength training. But bear in mind that this is advanced work.

Descriptions of Lifts

Focus Lifts

Power Clean (Hang position)

With your hands roughly shoulder width apart and using an overhand grip, lift the bar from the floor and stand upright to start the movement. From this position, push your hips back. The bar will move to the neutral position, in which your back is roughly at a 45 degree angle. (This is the safest posture for your back.) As the bar touches your knees, start the lift. Drive the bar upward (known as the *second pull*) by driving your hips through and rebending your knees (known as the *double-knee bend*). Continue to thrust upward, extending your ankles, knees, and hips (known as *triple extension*). Catch the bar on the fronts of your shoulders as you drop under it and perform a squat dip.

With your hands roughly shoulder width apart and using an overhand grip, lift the bar from the floor and stand upright to start the movement.

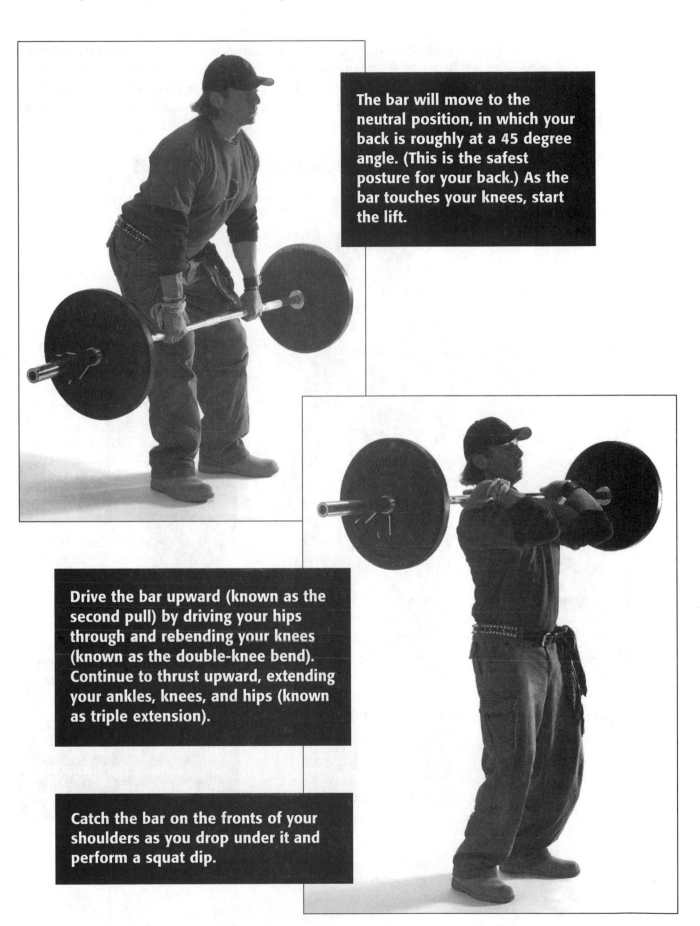

The bar will move to the neutral position, in which your back is roughly at a 45 degree angle. (This is the safest posture for your back.) As the bar touches your knees, start the lift.

Drive the bar upward (known as the second pull) by driving your hips through and rebending your knees (known as the double-knee bend). Continue to thrust upward, extending your ankles, knees, and hips (known as triple extension).

Catch the bar on the fronts of your shoulders as you drop under it and perform a squat dip.

Notes: Be patient as you learn this lift, and don't be in a rush to use a heavy load. And here's a special option for surfers: Instead of landing in a squat position, jump into a split lunge and then stand back up. Try to land your split such that your feet are roughly the same distance apart as would be the case when you pop up.

Power Clean (Hang position) on Swiss Ball

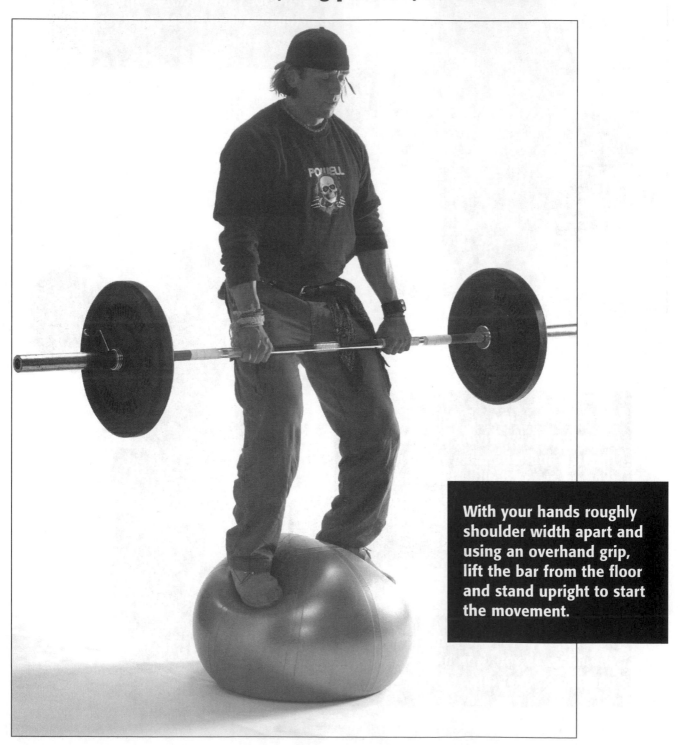

With your hands roughly shoulder width apart and using an overhand grip, lift the bar from the floor and stand upright to start the movement.

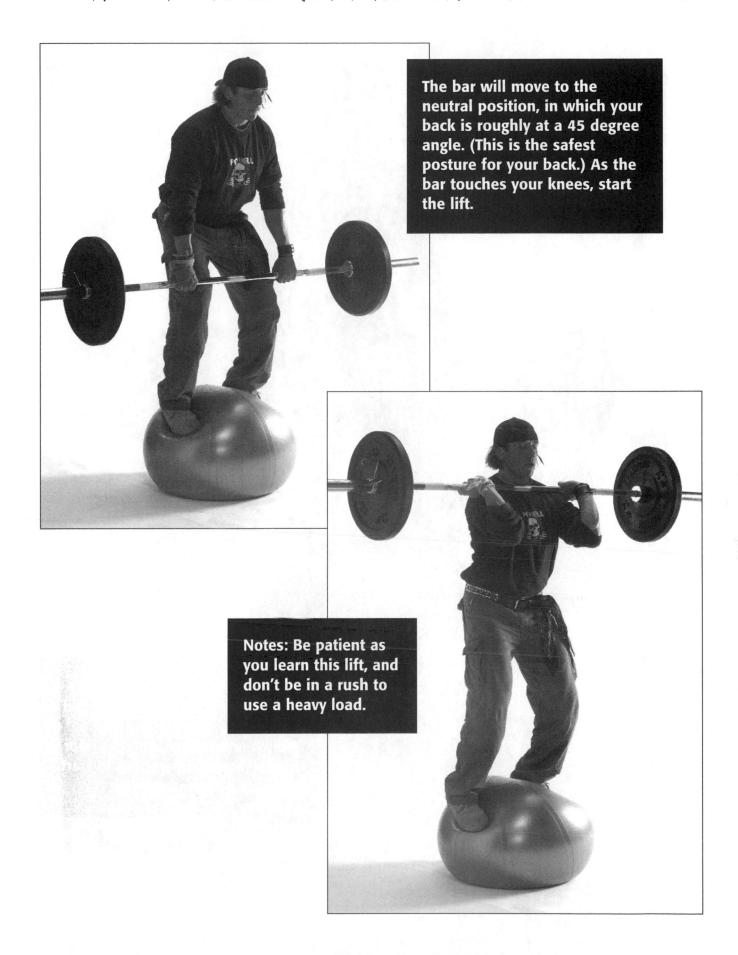

The bar will move to the neutral position, in which your back is roughly at a 45 degree angle. (This is the safest posture for your back.) As the bar touches your knees, start the lift.

Notes: Be patient as you learn this lift, and don't be in a rush to use a heavy load.

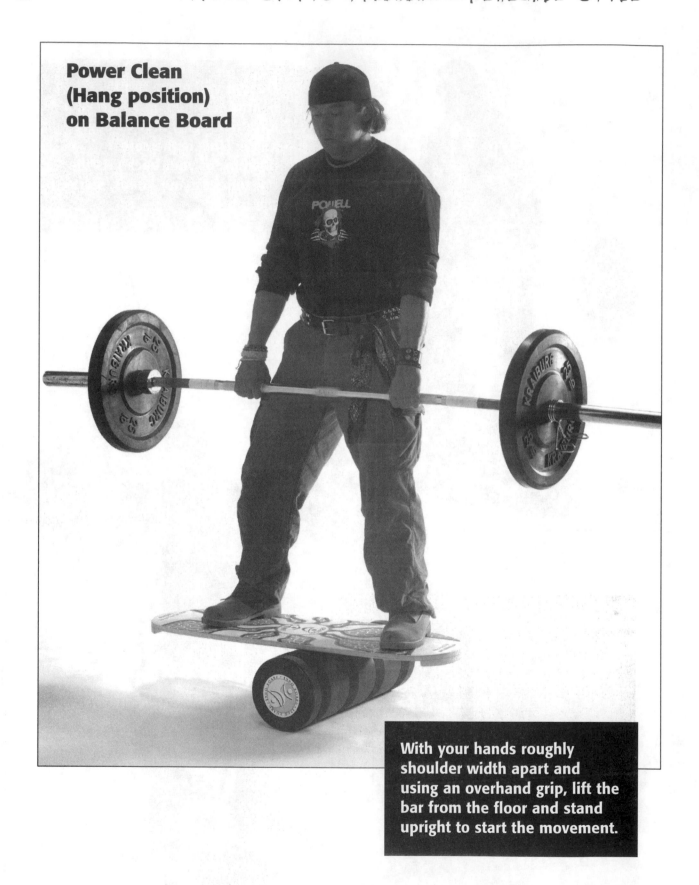

**Power Clean
(Hang position)
on Balance Board**

With your hands roughly shoulder width apart and using an overhand grip, lift the bar from the floor and stand upright to start the movement.

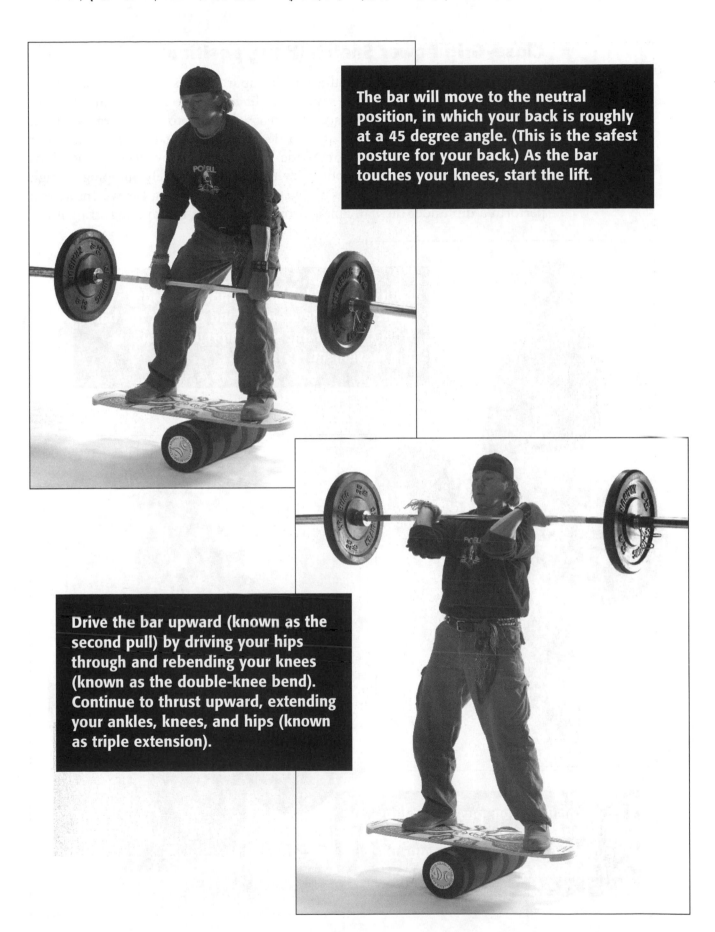

The bar will move to the neutral position, in which your back is roughly at a 45 degree angle. (This is the safest posture for your back.) As the bar touches your knees, start the lift.

Drive the bar upward (known as the second pull) by driving your hips through and rebending your knees (known as the double-knee bend). Continue to thrust upward, extending your ankles, knees, and hips (known as triple extension).

Close-Grip Power Snatch (Hang position)

With your hands roughly shoulder width apart and using an overhand grip, lift the bar from the floor and stand upright to initiate the movement. From this position, push your hips back. The bar will move to the neutral position, in which your back is roughly at a 45 degree angle. (Again, this is the safest posture for your back.) Next, explode the weight up by driving your hips forward and fully extending your body upward—effectively, jumping as high as possible. Lock out your arms above your head, catching the weight as you perform a dip under the bar. Finally, complete the lift by standing straight up.

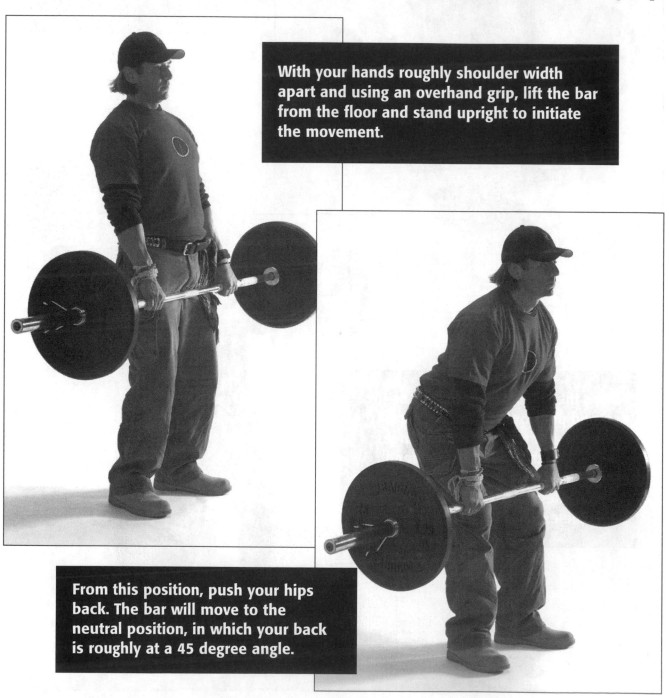

With your hands roughly shoulder width apart and using an overhand grip, lift the bar from the floor and stand upright to initiate the movement.

From this position, push your hips back. The bar will move to the neutral position, in which your back is roughly at a 45 degree angle.

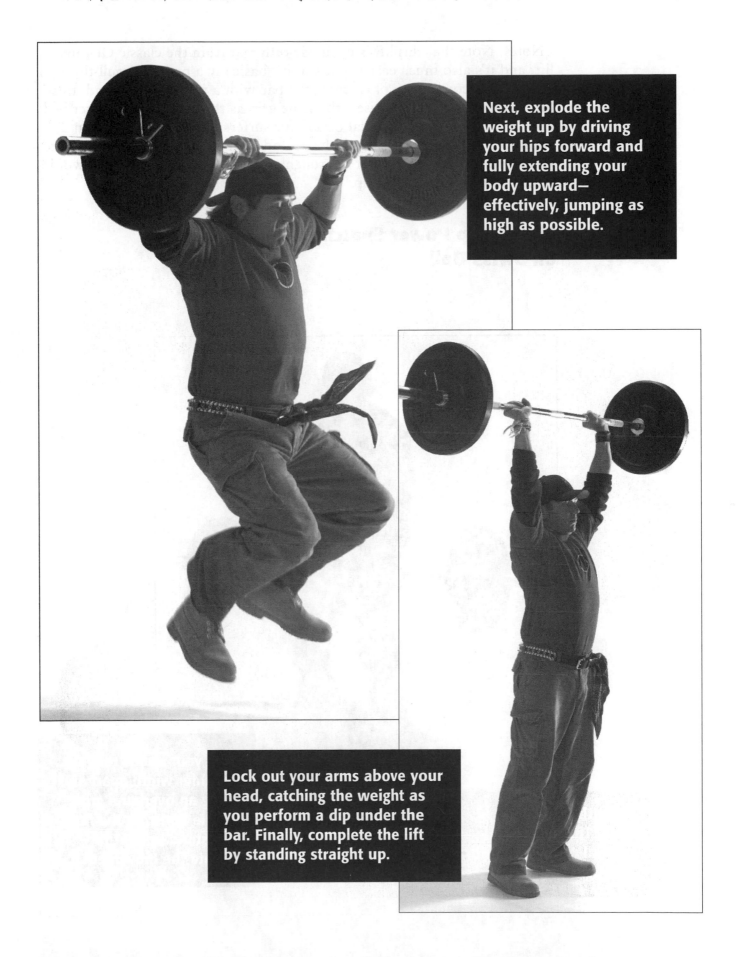

Next, explode the weight up by driving your hips forward and fully extending your body upward—effectively, jumping as high as possible.

Lock out your arms above your head, catching the weight as you perform a dip under the bar. Finally, complete the lift by standing straight up.

Notes: Note that this lift is distinctly different from the classic Olympic lift, and it's also much easier to learn. It's basically a powerful pull-through without the complexity of catching the bar with a wide grip. Instead, this lift is completed with precisely the same grip as the power clean (described above). Again, here's a special option for surfers: Instead of landing in a squat position, jump into a split lunge and then stand back up. Try to land your split such that your feet are roughly the same distance apart as would be the case when you pop up.

Close-Grip Power Snatch (Hang position) on Swiss Ball

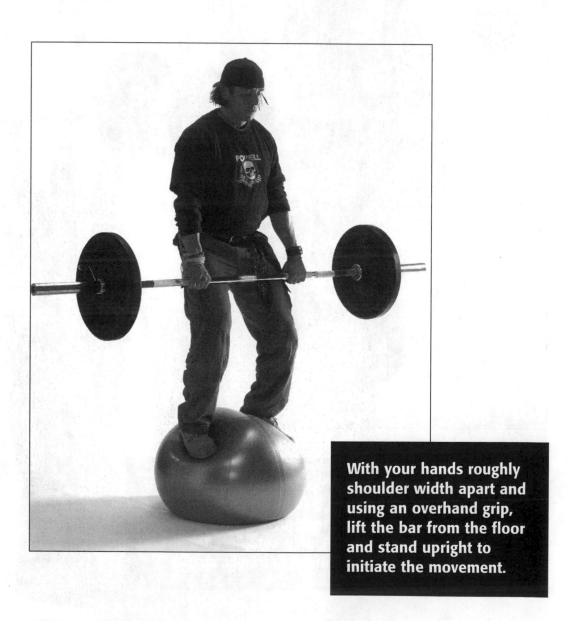

With your hands roughly shoulder width apart and using an overhand grip, lift the bar from the floor and stand upright to initiate the movement.

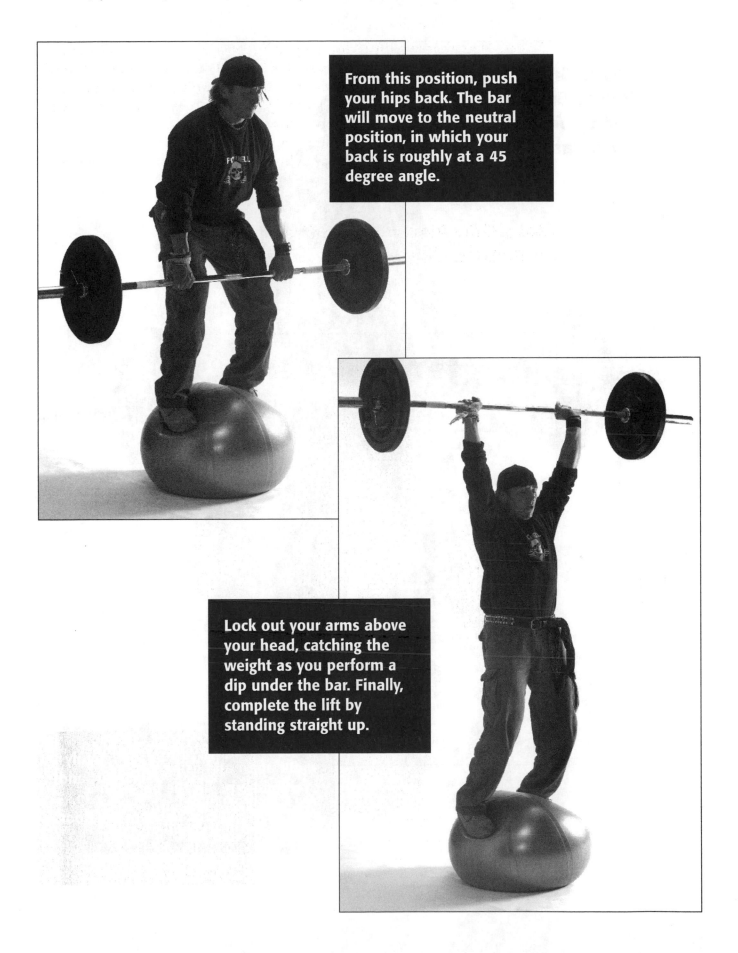

From this position, push your hips back. The bar will move to the neutral position, in which your back is roughly at a 45 degree angle.

Lock out your arms above your head, catching the weight as you perform a dip under the bar. Finally, complete the lift by standing straight up.

**Close-Grip
Power Snatch
(Hang position)
on Balance Board**

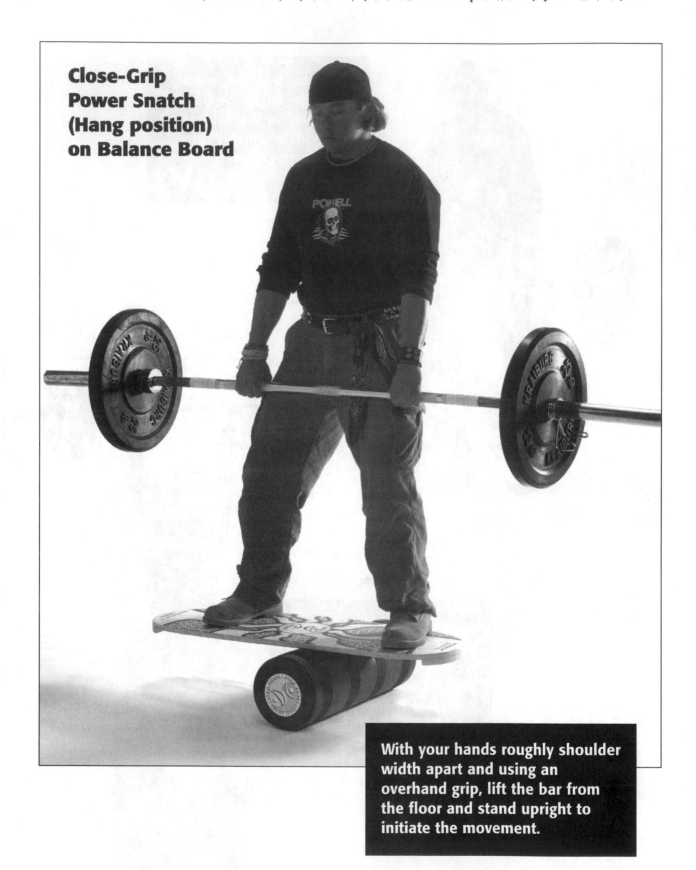

With your hands roughly shoulder width apart and using an overhand grip, lift the bar from the floor and stand upright to initiate the movement.

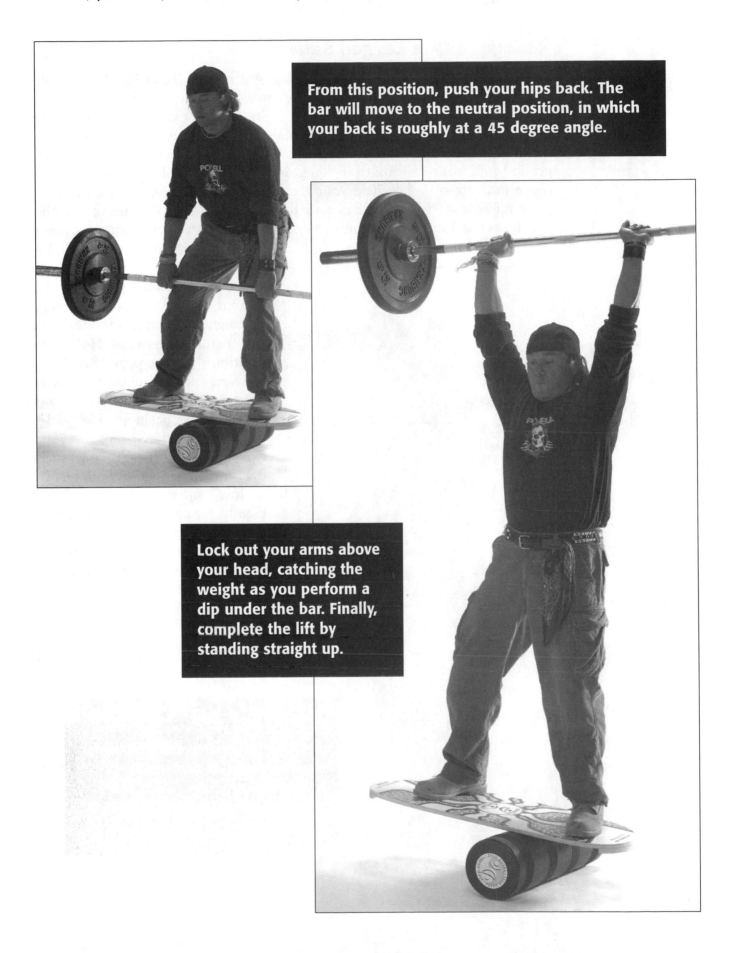

From this position, push your hips back. The bar will move to the neutral position, in which your back is roughly at a 45 degree angle.

Lock out your arms above your head, catching the weight as you perform a dip under the bar. Finally, complete the lift by standing straight up.

Renegade One-Legged Squat

This movement, never seen before, is one of most difficult lifts I have ever developed. It's a standard one-legged squat with a series of 15- to 30-second holds of different positions. The arms should be extended to the sides throughout the movement to help maintain balance. From a standing position (position 1), raise one leg such that your hip-to-knee joint is parallel to the ground and your calf and foot hang directly down. Hold this position. To move into position 2, extend your leg forward and straighten it; make sure your raised foot is perpendicular to the ground. Hold. (Be sure to breathe deeply, as the duration of the movement will likely start to tax your resources.)

Now move to position 3 by simultaneously swinging your raised leg back and extending your toe out as far as possible, creating a straight plane of head to toe that runs parallel to ground. Hold. For position 4, bring your knee back forward and extend your leg (as in position 2), squatting down into a rock-bottom position. Hold. To move to position 5, recoil your extended leg beneath you, such that you are sitting on both feet in a low squat position. Hold. Finally, for position 6, extend your opposite leg and squat upward. Repeat this entire series of positions and holds with the opposite leg.

Be sure to breathe deeply, as the duration of the movement will likely start to tax your resources.

Notes: Be patient with this maneuver, as it's quite taxing. For many, this will be a workout all on its own. Also be sure to breathe deeply throughout. Then, once you've mastered the series of movements, press yourself even further by doing the whole thing with your eyes closed. This will really push your balance!

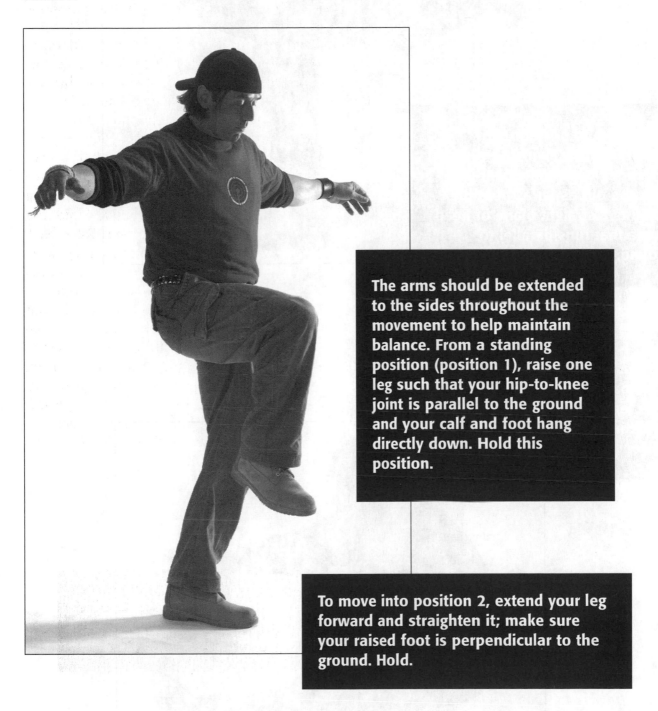

The arms should be extended to the sides throughout the movement to help maintain balance. From a standing position (position 1), raise one leg such that your hip-to-knee joint is parallel to the ground and your calf and foot hang directly down. Hold this position.

To move into position 2, extend your leg forward and straighten it; make sure your raised foot is perpendicular to the ground. Hold.

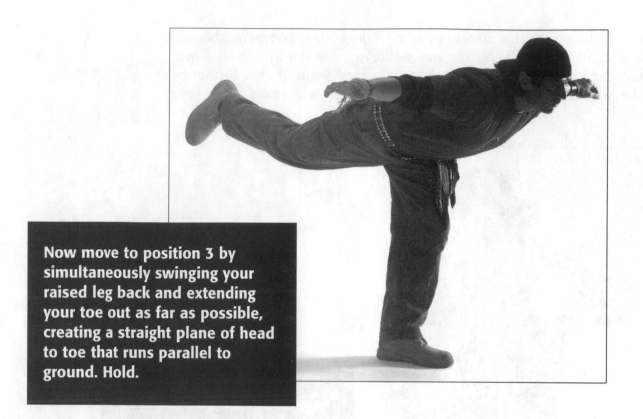

Now move to position 3 by simultaneously swinging your raised leg back and extending your toe out as far as possible, creating a straight plane of head to toe that runs parallel to ground. Hold.

For position 4, bring your knee back forward and extend your leg (as in position 2), squatting down into a rock-bottom position. Hold.

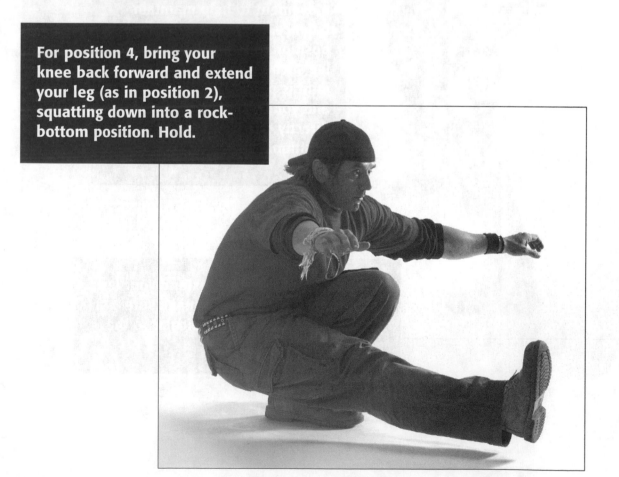

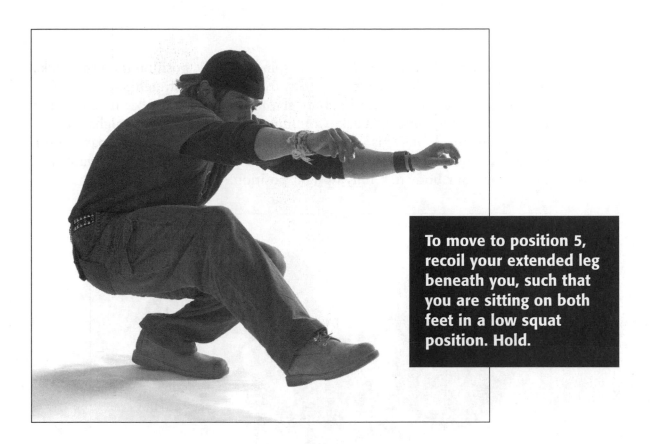

To move to position 5, recoil your extended leg beneath you, such that you are sitting on both feet in a low squat position. Hold.

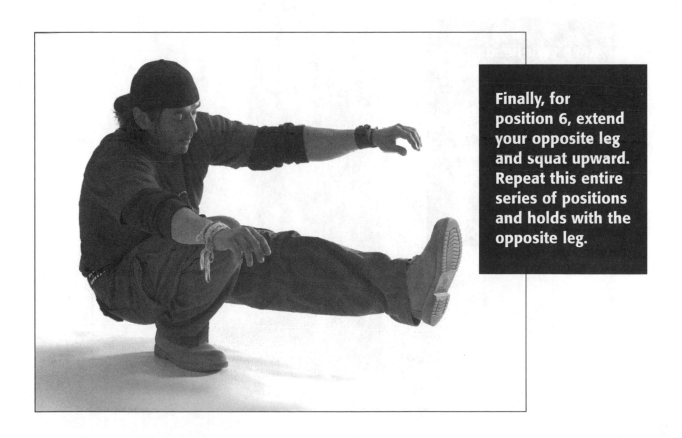

Finally, for position 6, extend your opposite leg and squat upward. Repeat this entire series of positions and holds with the opposite leg.

Squat

Take the barbell from a rack, and grasping it firmly, position it on the backs of your shoulders. Keep your head forward, your back straight, and your feet flat on the floor. With your feet about shoulder width apart, begin descending by pushing your buttocks back. Continue to squat until your thighs are just past parallel to floor. (This will likely take some practice.) Once at parallel (or as low as you can go), push the bar up by thrusting your hips forward and extending your body to a fully upright position.

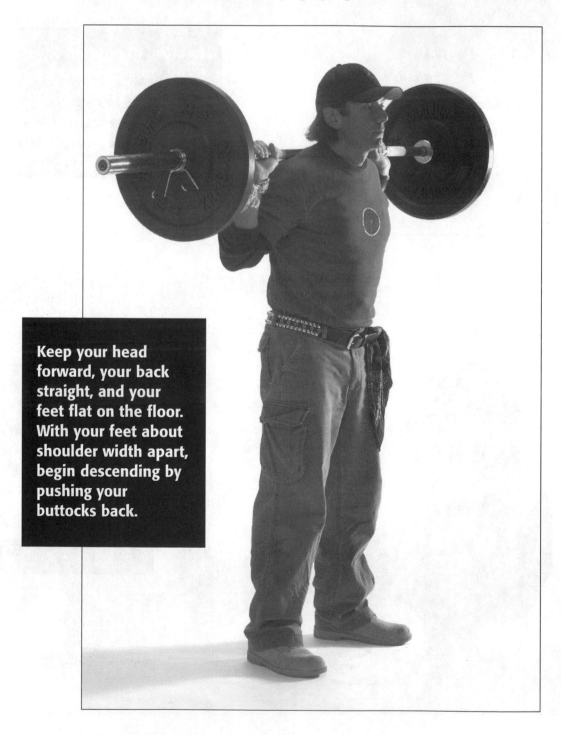

Keep your head forward, your back straight, and your feet flat on the floor. With your feet about shoulder width apart, begin descending by pushing your buttocks back.

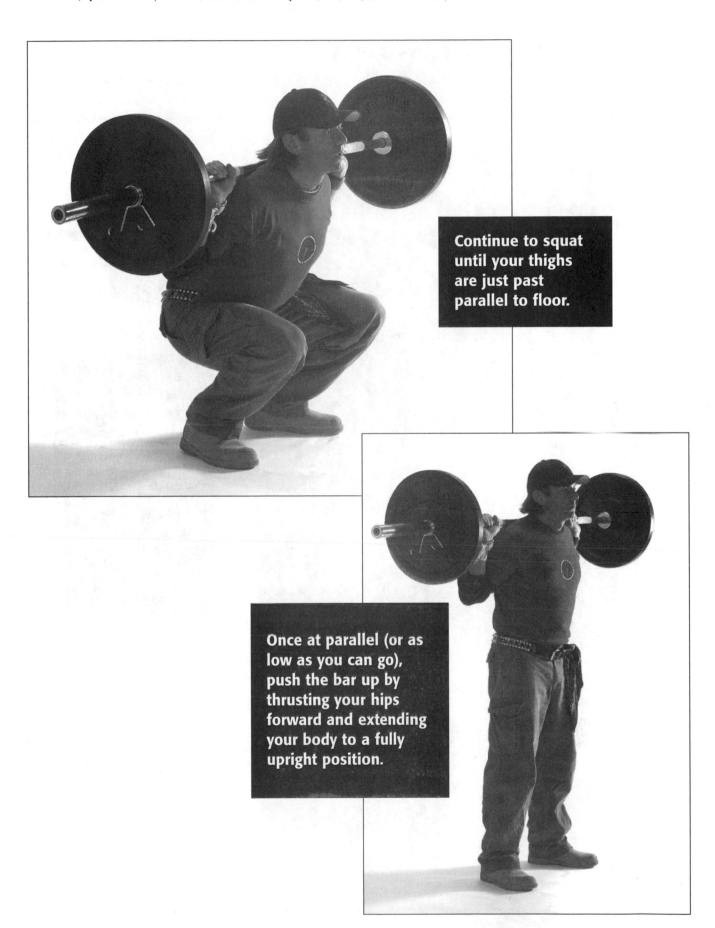

Continue to squat until your thighs are just past parallel to floor.

Once at parallel (or as low as you can go), push the bar up by thrusting your hips forward and extending your body to a fully upright position.

Squat on Swiss Ball

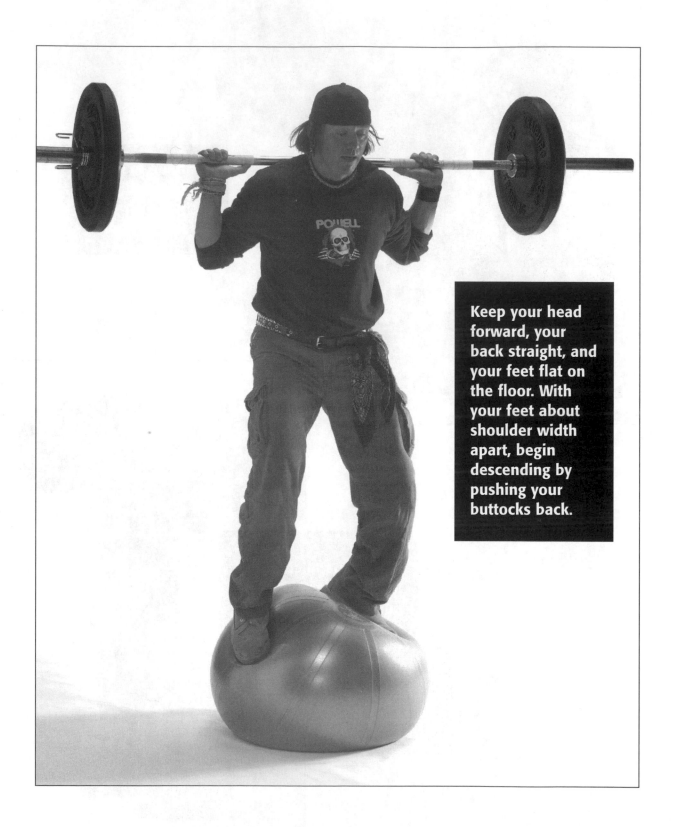

Keep your head forward, your back straight, and your feet flat on the floor. With your feet about shoulder width apart, begin descending by pushing your buttocks back.

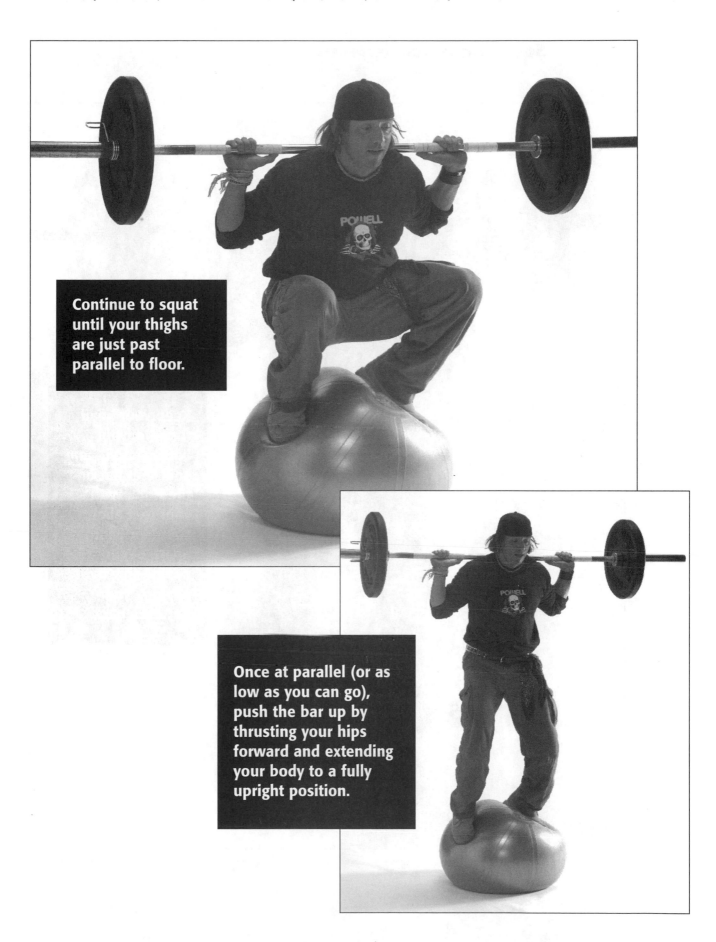

Continue to squat until your thighs are just past parallel to floor.

Once at parallel (or as low as you can go), push the bar up by thrusting your hips forward and extending your body to a fully upright position.

Squat on Balance Board

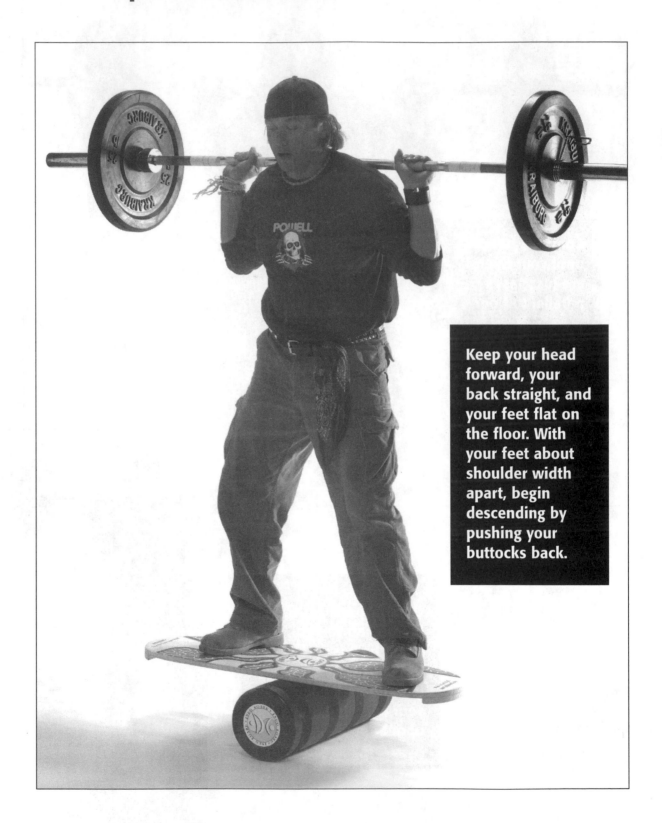

Keep your head forward, your back straight, and your feet flat on the floor. With your feet about shoulder width apart, begin descending by pushing your buttocks back.

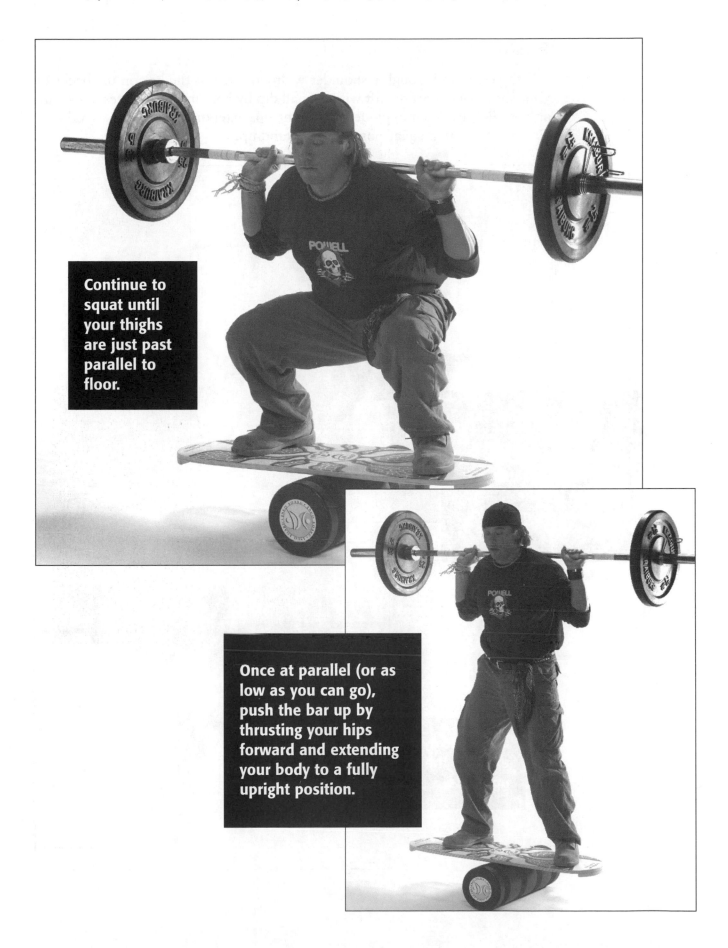

Continue to squat until your thighs are just past parallel to floor.

Once at parallel (or as low as you can go), push the bar up by thrusting your hips forward and extending your body to a fully upright position.

Push Jerk

With your hands roughly shoulder width apart, rest the bar on the backs of your shoulders. Start the lift with a small dip by bending your knees, hips, and ankles slightly. Then explode the weight up, extending your arms overhead. Catch the bar in a squat position and stand up.

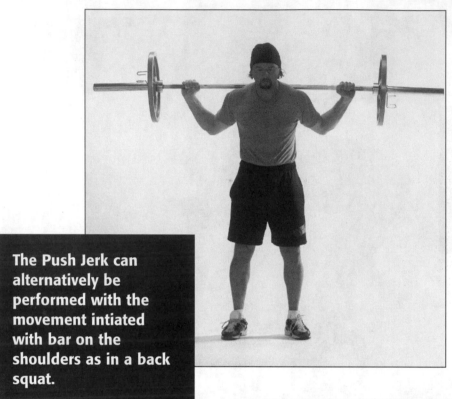

The Push Jerk can alternatively be performed with the movement intiated with bar on the shoulders as in a back squat.

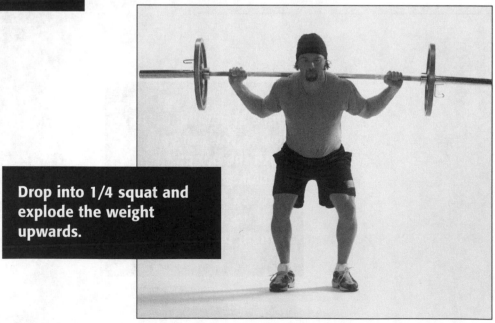

Drop into 1/4 squat and explode the weight upwards.

Notes: Overhead movements are tremendously effective and satisfy many training needs, but all too often, athletes injure themselves in doing these movements because they go too heavy. Don't make that mistake. Use a safe training load. Again, here's an option for surfers: Instead of landing in a squat position, jump into a split lunge and then stand back up. Try to land your split such that your feet are roughly the same distance apart as would be the case when you pop up.

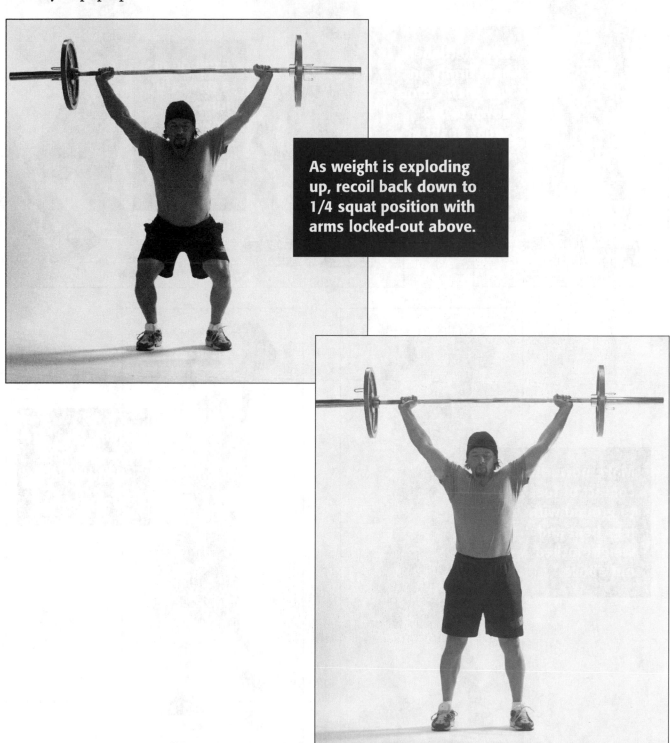

As weight is exploding up, recoil back down to 1/4 squat position with arms locked-out above.

Push Jerk with Kettlebells

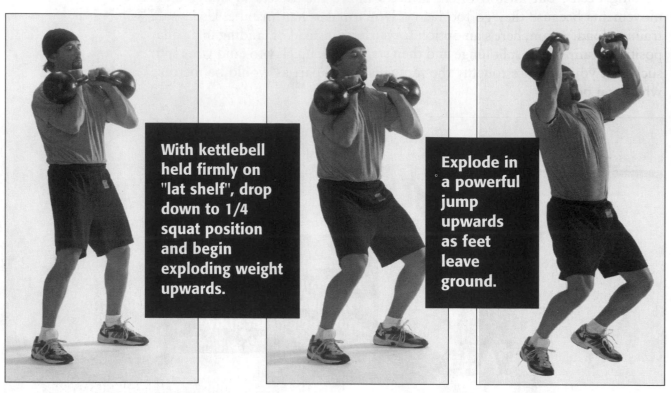

With kettlebell held firmly on "lat shelf", drop down to 1/4 squat position and begin exploding weight upwards.

Explode in a powerful jump upwards as feet leave ground.

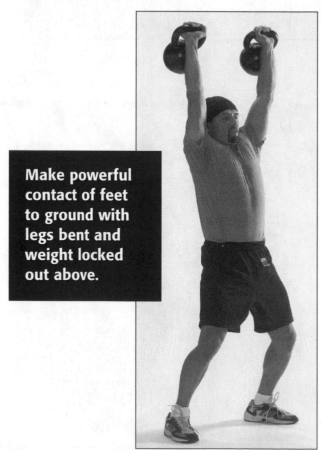

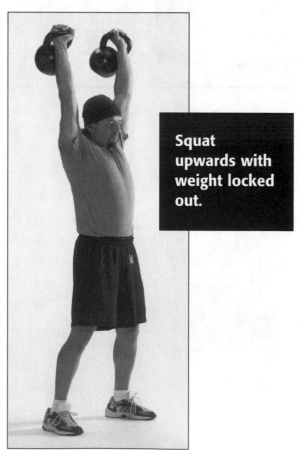

Make powerful contact of feet to ground with legs bent and weight locked out above.

Squat upwards with weight locked out.

Bench Press

Begin in a supine position, lying on a bench with the barbell in a rack just above your chest at about nipple level. Your feet should start and then remain flat on the floor. Grasp the bar with your hands roughly shoulder-width apart, pinching together your rear deltoids. Disengage the bar from the rack and lower it to your chest. Keep your elbows in tight and maintain control; don't bounce. As the bar touches your chest, drive it up in an explosive manner.

Notes: Change the width of your grip often in order to prevent adaptation to a specific range of motion. A tremendous option with this lift is to perform it while lying on a Swiss ball. Doing so will ensure retraction of the shoulders.

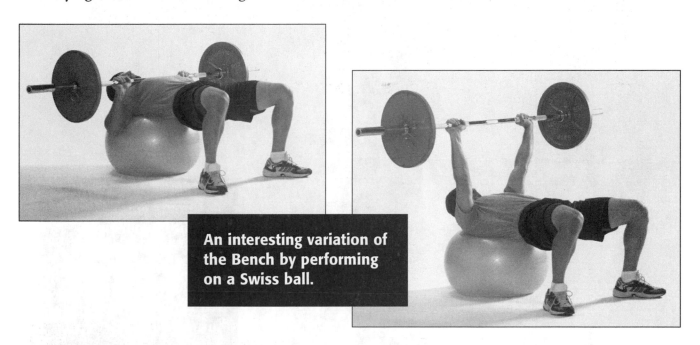

An interesting variation of the Bench by performing on a Swiss ball.

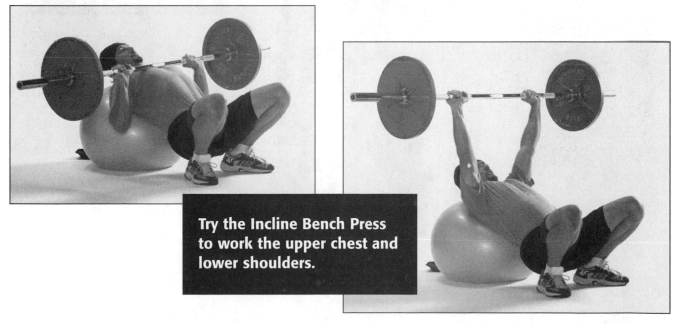

Try the Incline Bench Press to work the upper chest and lower shoulders.

Bent Press

Assuming you have the weight in your right hand, position your feet slightly more than shoulder width apart with your left foot turned out. Extend your right arm straight out and hold the weight at shoulder height with your palm facing in. To begin, make a corkscrew movement underneath and to the side, and turning your hand clockwise and upward. When your hand is extended completely up and you are bent over, straighten up.

Notes: This movement can be performed with either a barbell or a kettlebell. If you use a barbell, be aware that the turning of the bar makes the lift that more challenging. The set up is important.

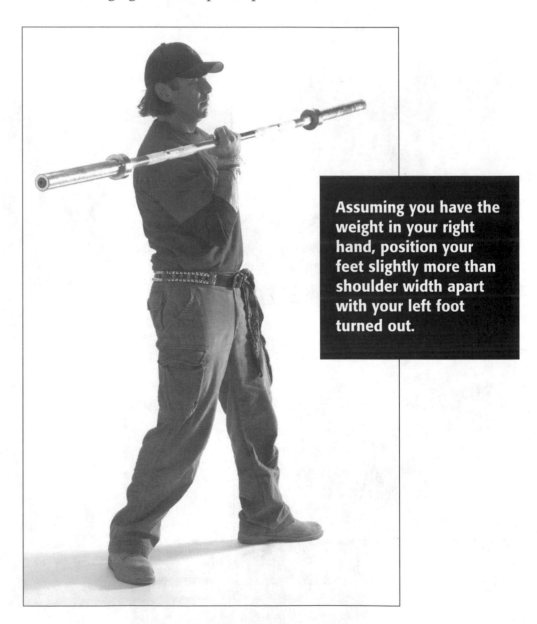

Assuming you have the weight in your right hand, position your feet slightly more than shoulder width apart with your left foot turned out.

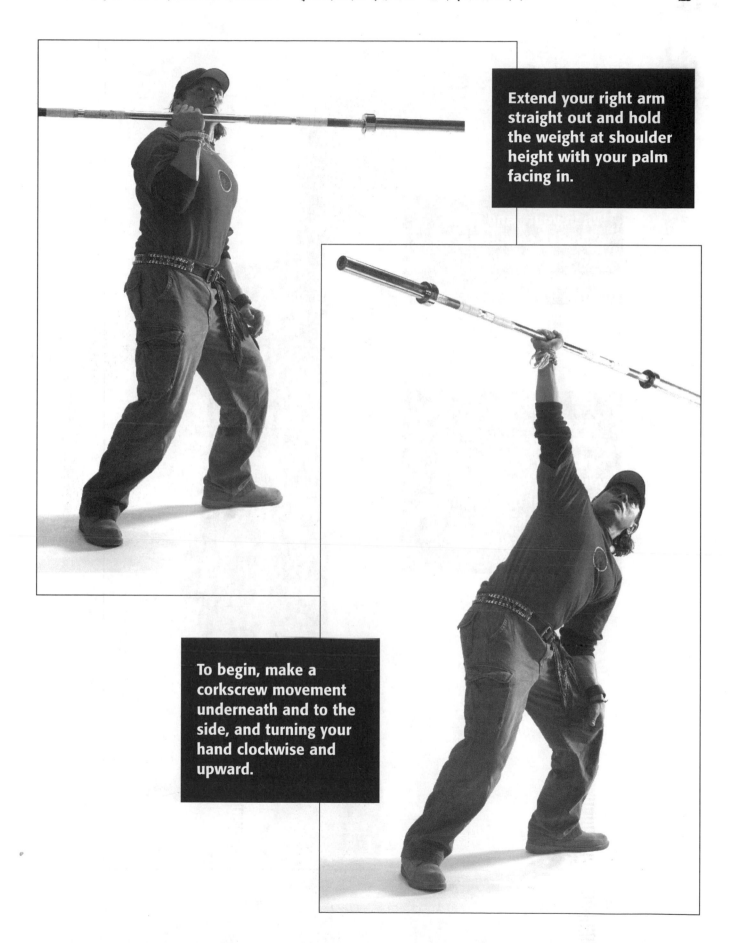

Extend your right arm straight out and hold the weight at shoulder height with your palm facing in.

To begin, make a corkscrew movement underneath and to the side, and turning your hand clockwise and upward.

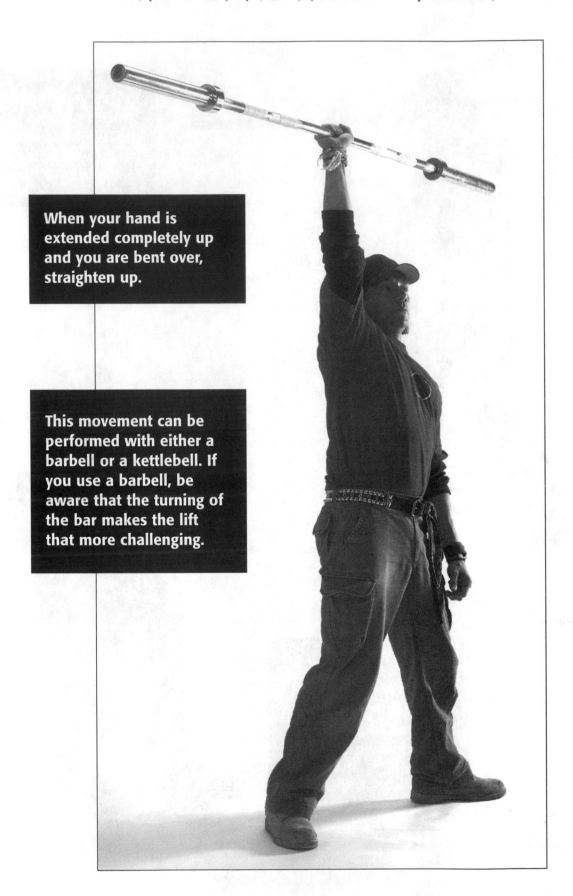

When your hand is extended completely up and you are bent over, straighten up.

This movement can be performed with either a barbell or a kettlebell. If you use a barbell, be aware that the turning of the bar makes the lift that more challenging.

Hybrid Lifts

One-Arm Power Clean

See the explanation of the "Power clean" in the previous section, and adapt the lift so as to use just one arm. Alternate arms, performing the same number of reps with each.

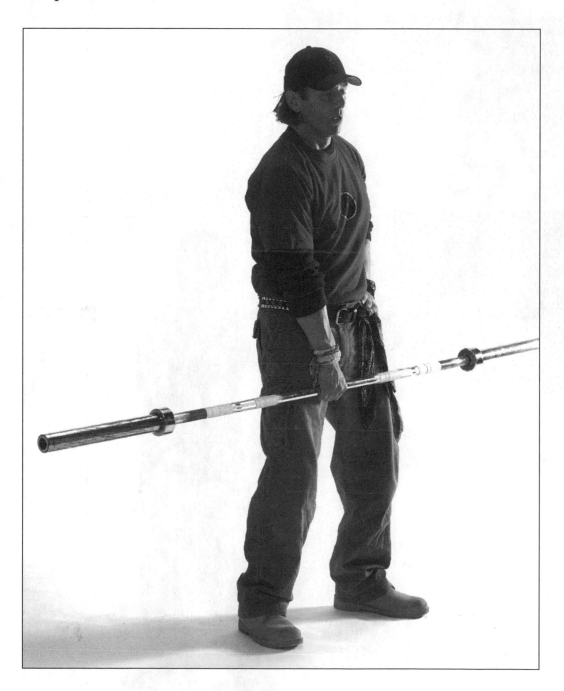

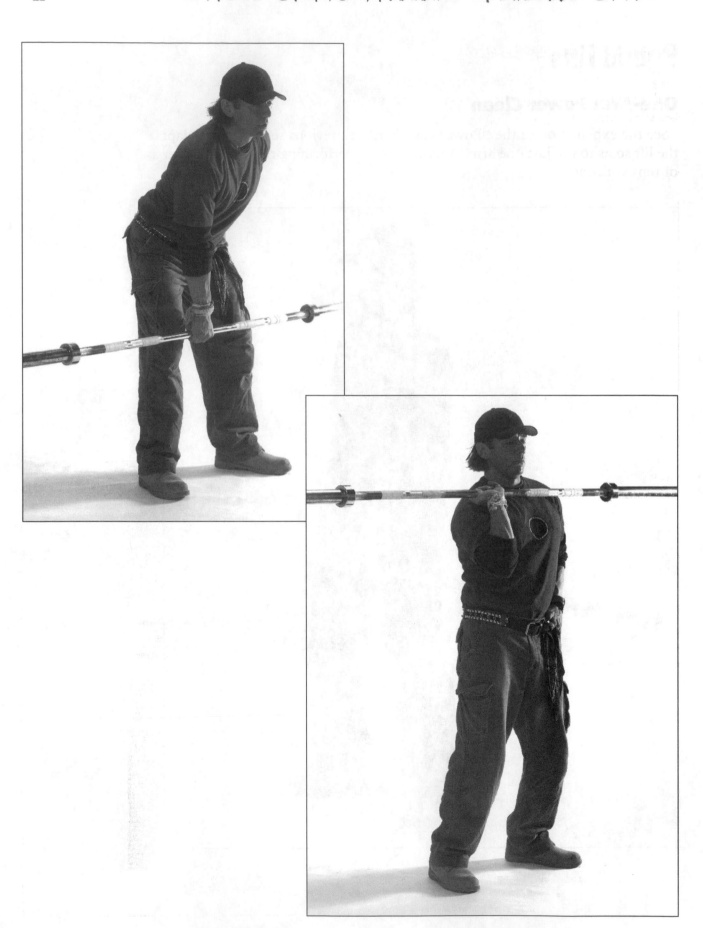

One-Arm Power Snatch

See the explanation of the "Close-grip power snatch" in the previous section, and adapt the lift so as to use just one arm. Alternate arms, performing the same number of reps with each.

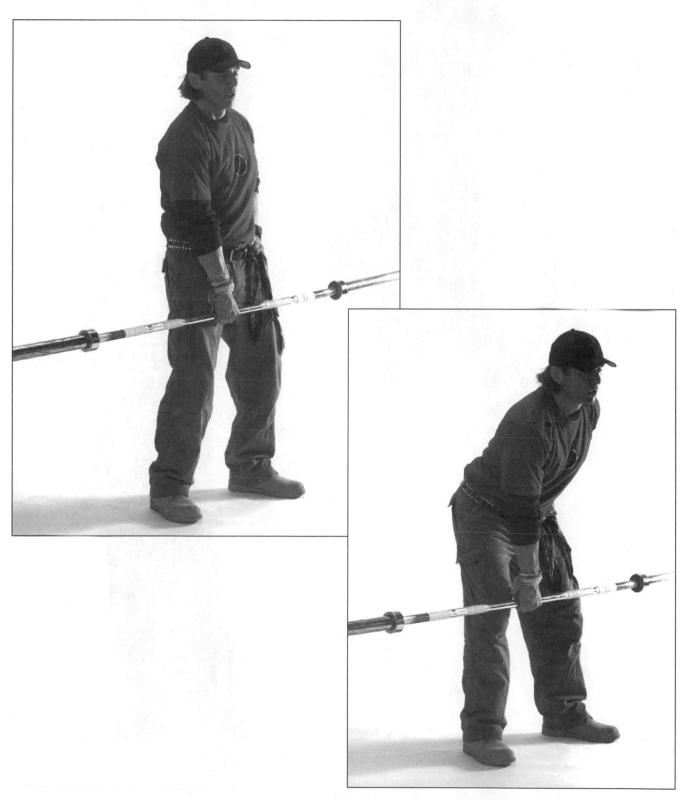

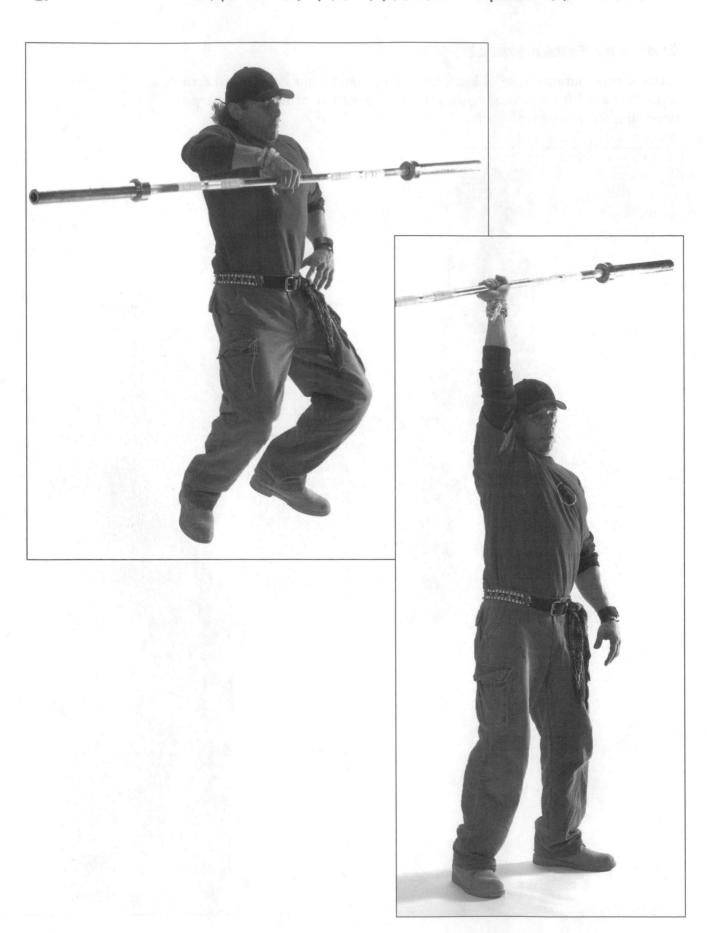

Crossover Kettlebell Snatch

This is one of my favorite movements, and it can be performed in two definite styles. (The first is not as advanced as the second.) In the initial style, begin with the kettlebell resting on the ground to the outside of your left foot. Then grasp the bell with your right hand, ensuring that your torso is turned such that your shoulders are nearly perpindicular to your feet. Pull the weight up as if you are executing a standard kettlebell snatch. In the second, more advanced style, place your left foot and the kettlebell on a box that's approximately 6 to 12 inches in height. (Again, the weight should be to the outside of your foot.) Complete the lift as you did the first style, but use your left to exert pressure on the box and assist in your drive.

Note: BMX and MTB riders will really feel the sport-specific benefits of doing this lift.

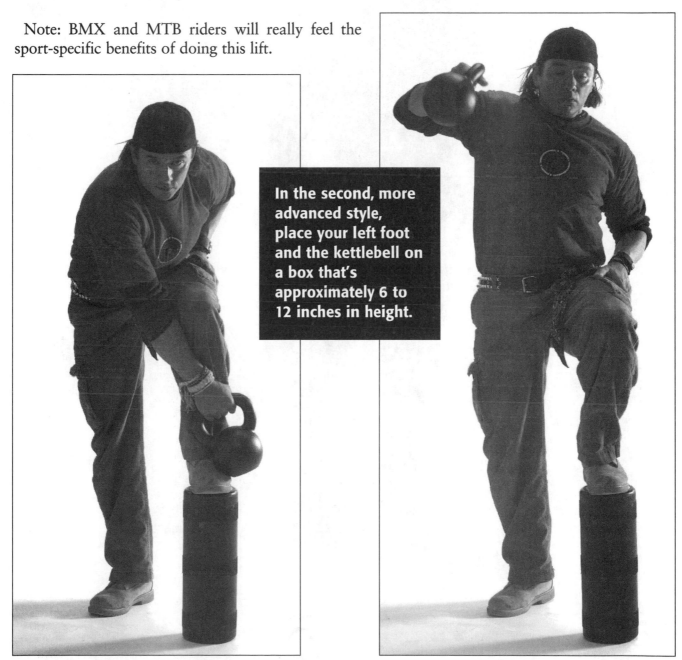

In the second, more advanced style, place your left foot and the kettlebell on a box that's approximately 6 to 12 inches in height.

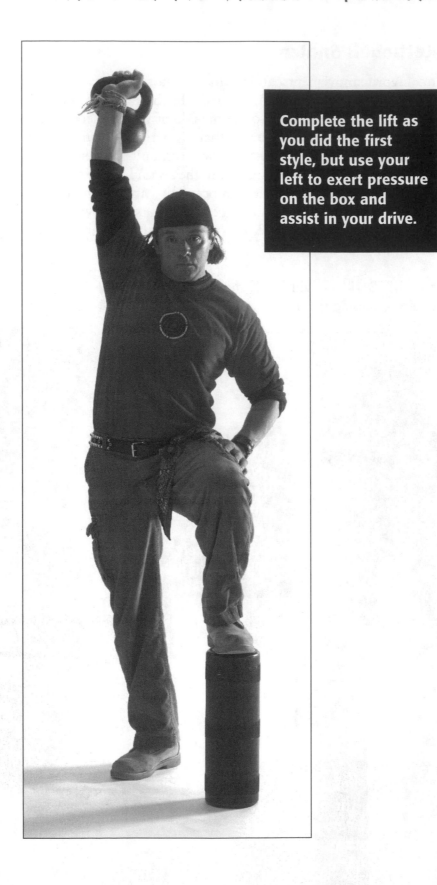

Complete the lift as you did the first style, but use your left to exert pressure on the box and assist in your drive.

Pipeline

Begin with your feet roughly 2 to 3 feet apart and turned out at 45 degreebangles. Bend your body to one side allowing the knee and shin of back leg to come to ground and turn your foot over. Be sure your lead foot stays flat on the ground throughout the movement. Lead hand stay in line with knee of lead foot.

Note this unique stretch has obvious roots in Surfing.

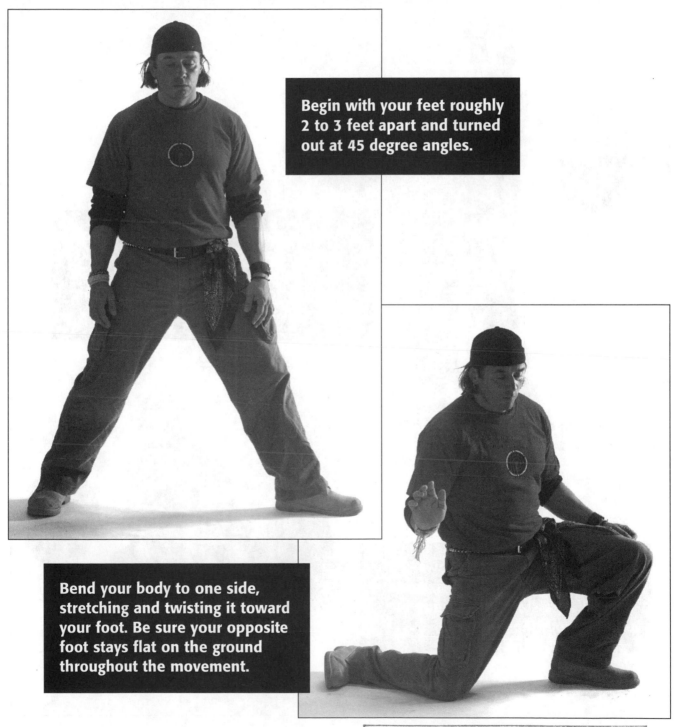

Begin with your feet roughly 2 to 3 feet apart and turned out at 45 degree angles.

Bend your body to one side, stretching and twisting it toward your foot. Be sure your opposite foot stays flat on the ground throughout the movement.

Zercher Squat

With your arms extended in front of you, palms up, position the bar in the crooks of your arms. Holding the bar in place, bring your forearms up, squeezing them tight against your body. Initiate the squatting movement by pushing your buttocks back and lowering your body. Squat down until your elbows touch your legs at midthigh. Raise yourself to a standing position by pushing your hips forward.

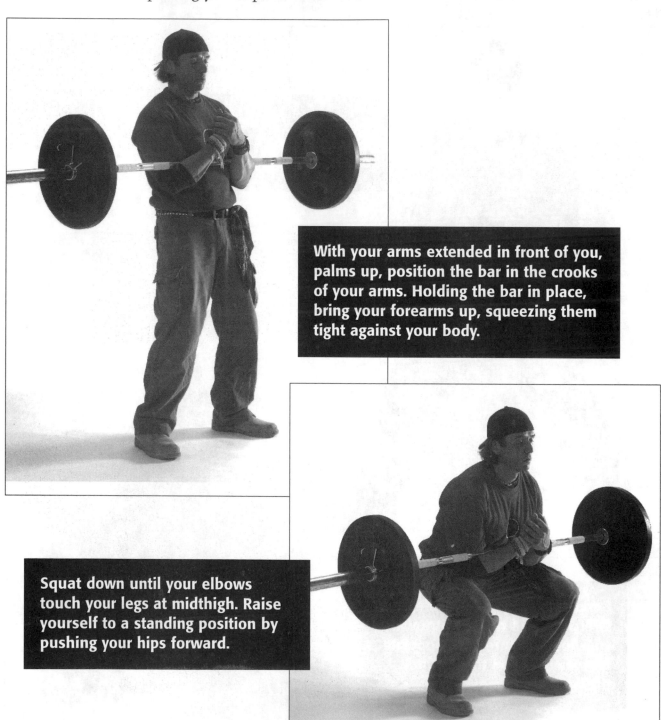

With your arms extended in front of you, palms up, position the bar in the crooks of your arms. Holding the bar in place, bring your forearms up, squeezing them tight against your body.

Squat down until your elbows touch your legs at midthigh. Raise yourself to a standing position by pushing your hips forward.

Front Squat

This is essentially a barbell squat in which the weight is distributed on your chest. Hold the bar in your hands in what's termed "the rack." To do so, hold your elbows up high, such that the line from your underarms to your elbows is at or near parallel to the ground. Begin to squat by pushing your buttocks back and lowering your body. Squat until your thighs are just below parallel to the ground. Push your hips forward to begin your ascent, and rise to a standing position.

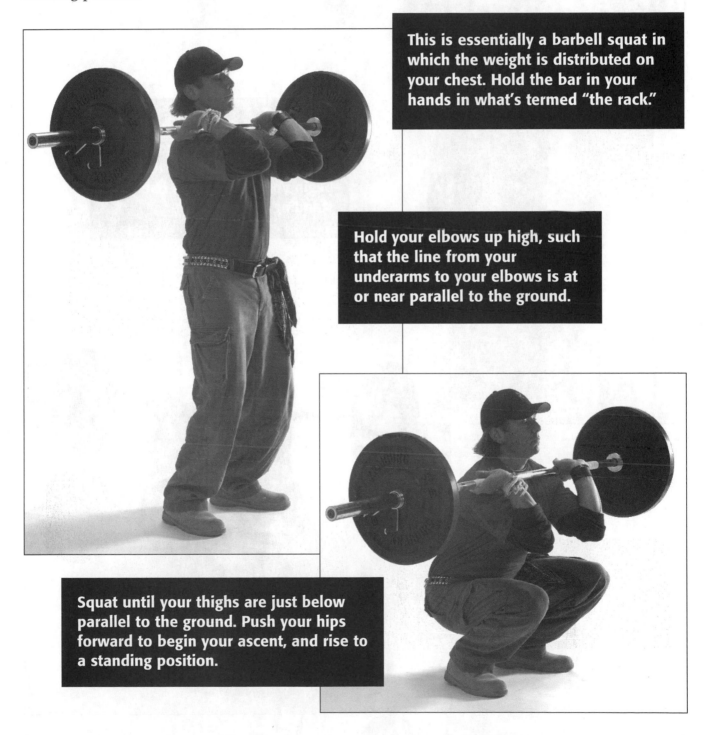

This is essentially a barbell squat in which the weight is distributed on your chest. Hold the bar in your hands in what's termed "the rack."

Hold your elbows up high, such that the line from your underarms to your elbows is at or near parallel to the ground.

Squat until your thighs are just below parallel to the ground. Push your hips forward to begin your ascent, and rise to a standing position.

Front Squat on Swiss Ball

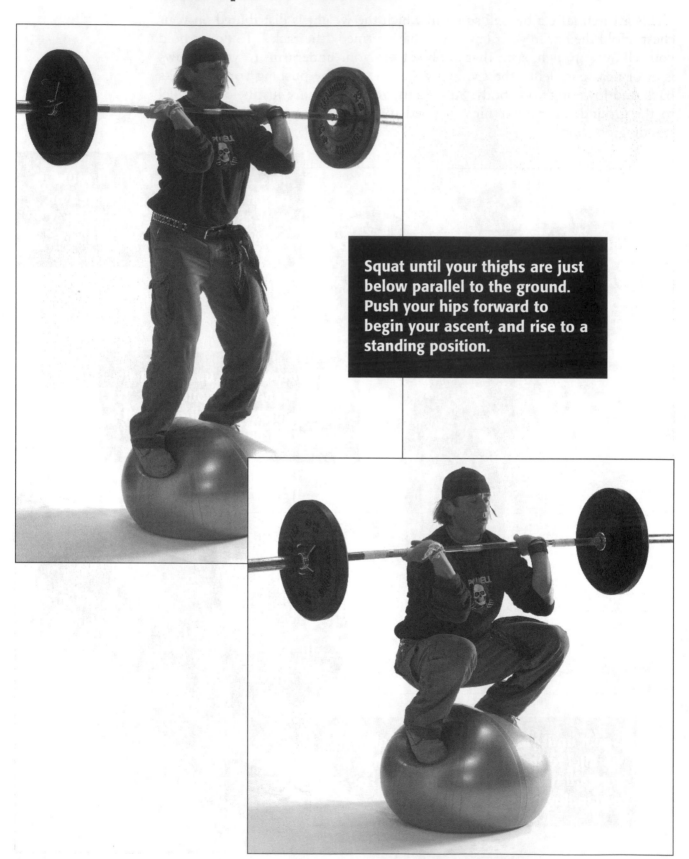

Squat until your thighs are just below parallel to the ground. Push your hips forward to begin your ascent, and rise to a standing position.

Front Squat on Balance Board

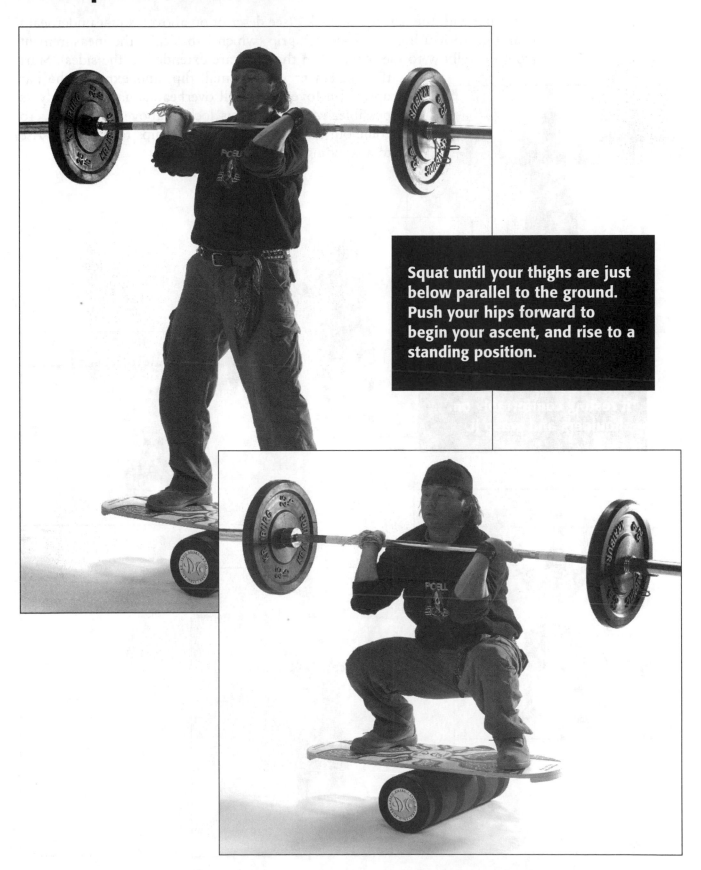

Squat until your thighs are just below parallel to the ground. Push your hips forward to begin your ascent, and rise to a standing position.

Drop Snatch

Starting with the bar in "the rack" (see description above), squat underneath it and grasp it using a wide-snatch grip (which is basically the measurement from one elbow to the other when the arms are extended to the sides). Start the movement with a small dip, and explode the bar upward. Move into a full overhead squat as quickly as possible, with your arms locked above your head. To come out of the squat, push your hips forward and rise to a standing position.

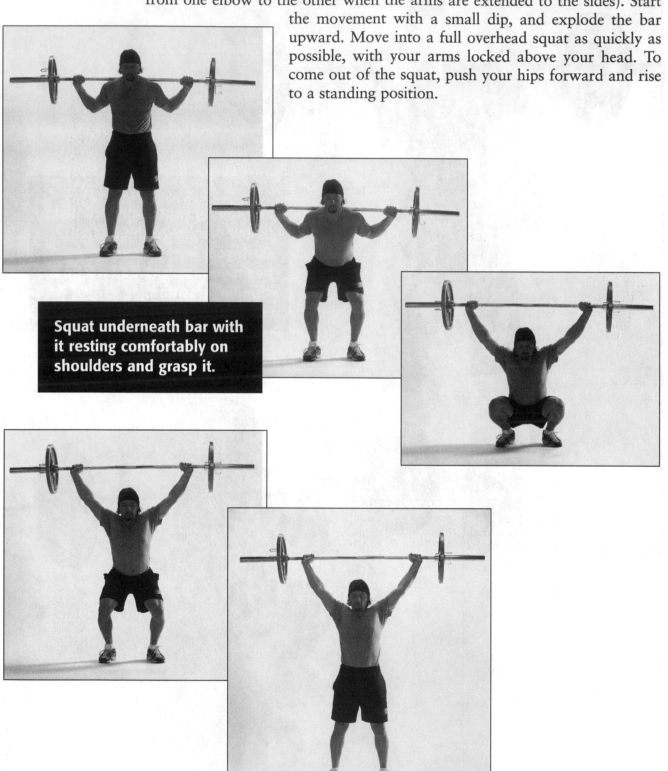

Squat underneath bar with it resting comfortably on shoulders and grasp it.

One-Arm Deadlift

With the weight on the ground, stand perpendicular to it. Bend down, keeping your back in a neutral position (or bent at about 45 degrees), and grasp the middle of the bar with one hand. Then lift the weight up and return to a standing position.

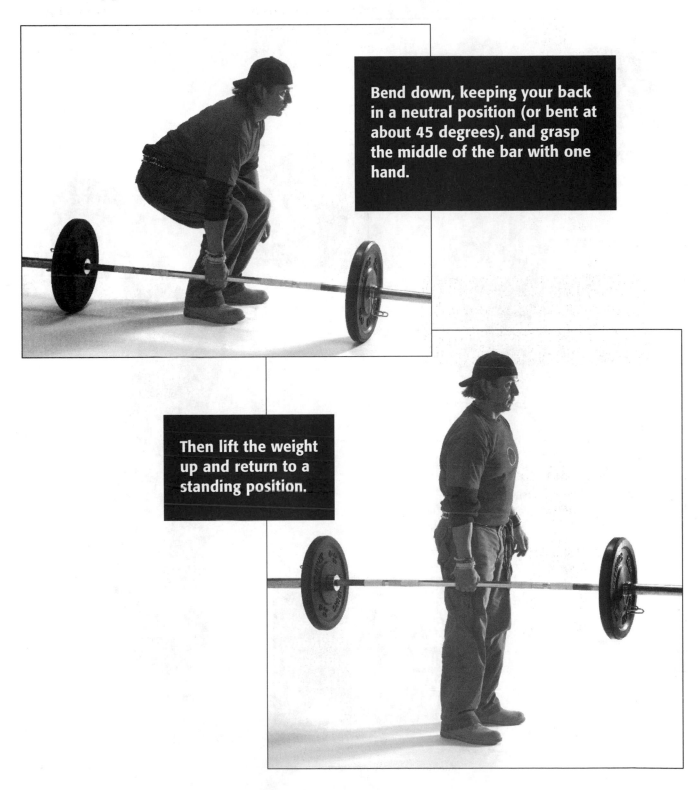

Bend down, keeping your back in a neutral position (or bent at about 45 degrees), and grasp the middle of the bar with one hand.

Then lift the weight up and return to a standing position.

Shoulder Press

This lift can be performed in a standing or a seated position and using barbells, dumbbells, kettlebells, or virtually any nonconforming object. Using an overhand, shoulder-width grip, press the bar overhead and then lower it again. Maintain control throughout the movement.

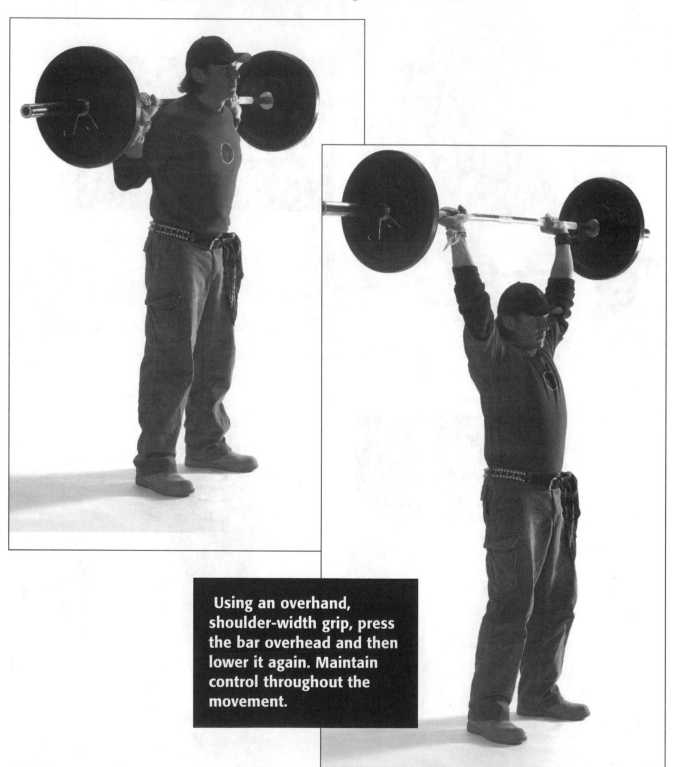

Using an overhand, shoulder-width grip, press the bar overhead and then lower it again. Maintain control throughout the movement.

Shoulder Press on Balance Board

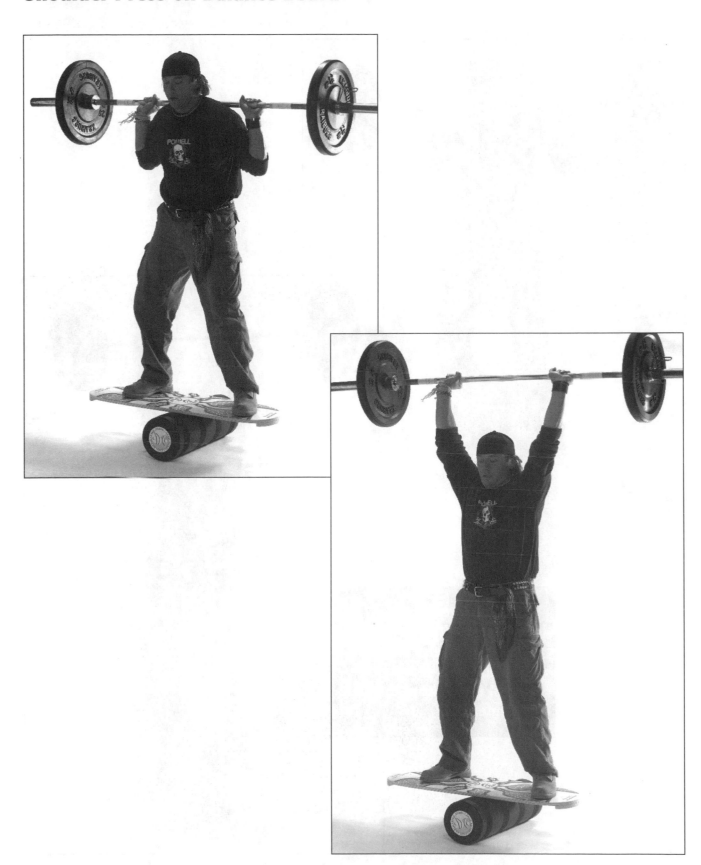

Shoulder Press on Balance Ball

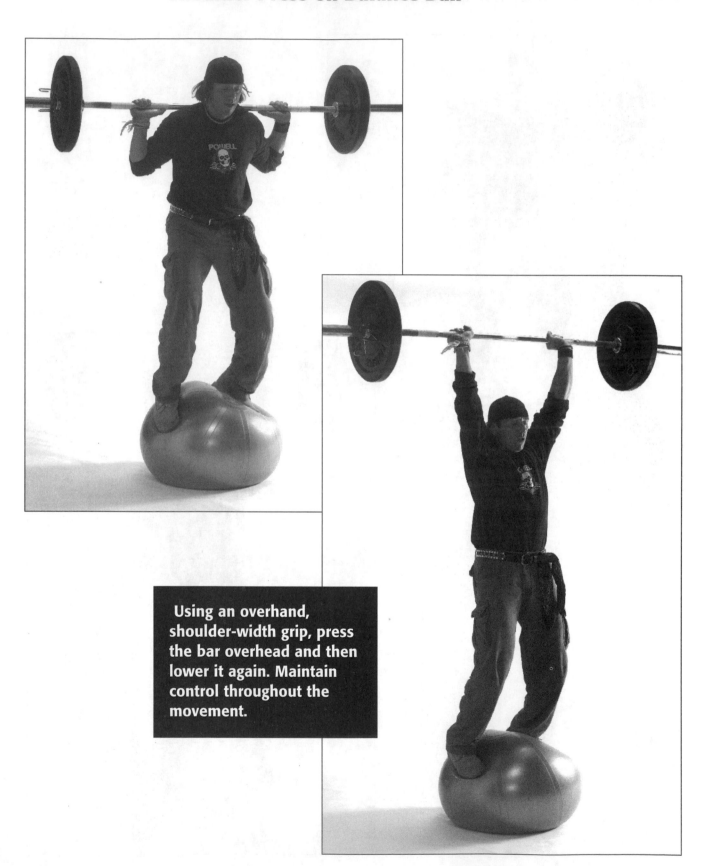

Using an overhand, shoulder-width grip, press the bar overhead and then lower it again. Maintain control throughout the movement.

Shoulder Press with Dumbells on Balance Ball

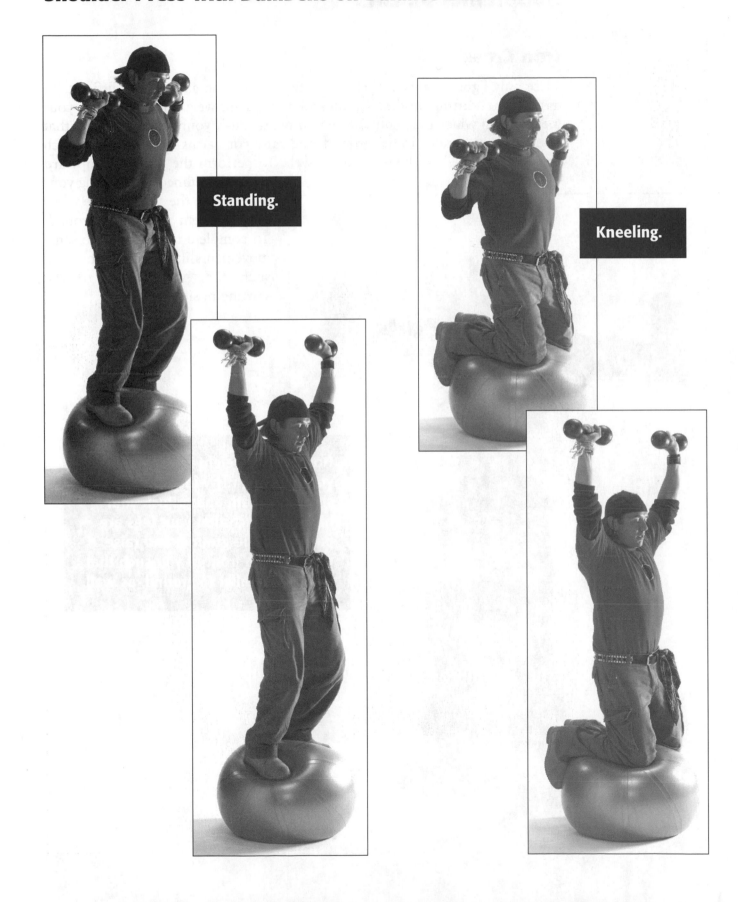

Standing.

Kneeling.

Supplemental Lifts

Iron Cross

Use only light weights in performing this movement, as it is very difficult. To assume the starting position, stand and hold a light weight in each hand, your feet slightly wider than shoulder width apart. Push your hips back such that your legs are parallel to the ground, and raise your arms in front of you such that they parallel to the ground, as well. To perform the lift, squat upward while simultaneously moving your arms out to the sides, all the while keeping them parallel to ground. To complete the lift, do the same movements in the opposite order, such that you return to the starting position.

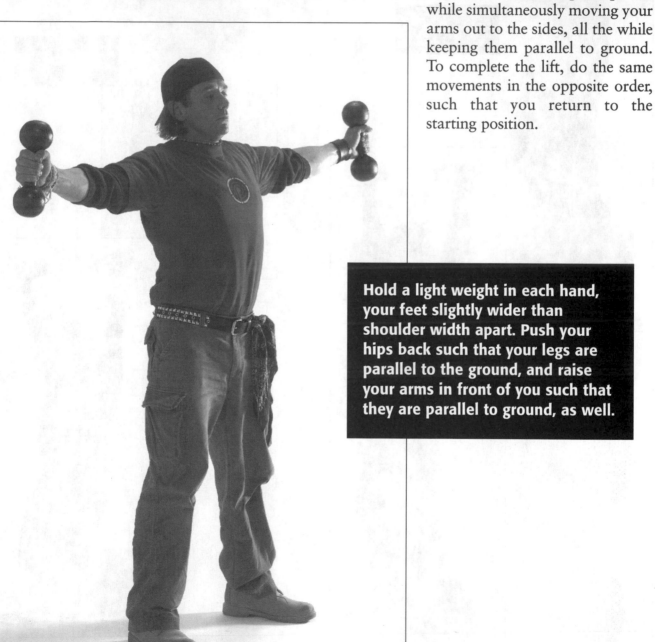

Hold a light weight in each hand, your feet slightly wider than shoulder width apart. Push your hips back such that your legs are parallel to the ground, and raise your arms in front of you such that they are parallel to ground, as well.

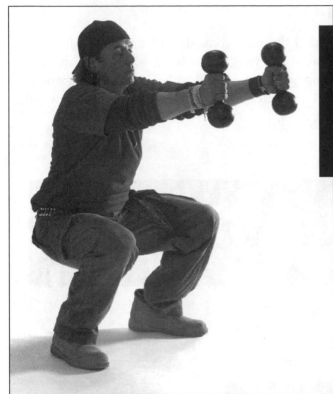

Squat upward while simultaneously moving your arms out to the sides, all the while keeping them parallel to ground. To complete the lift, do the same movements in the opposite order, such that you return to the starting position.

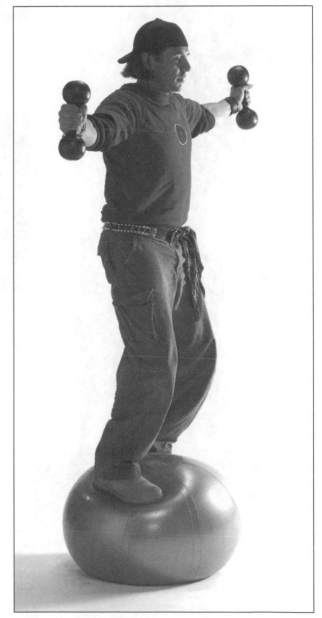

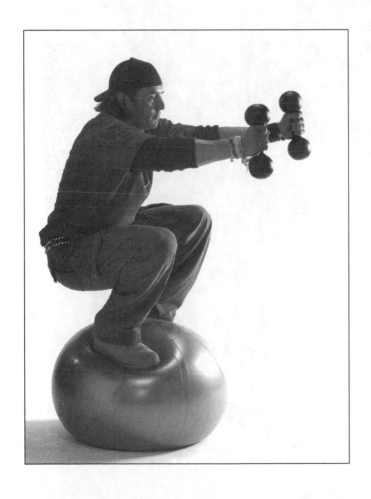

Renegade Squat-Pull

To start, stand with your feet slightly more than shoulder width apart. Grasp a kettlebell in each hand, and hold the weights in front of you at hip height. Intiate the movement by pushing your hips back and allowing the kettlebells to nearly touch ground. From this position, squat upward and pull the weights up, such that hands are at chest level.

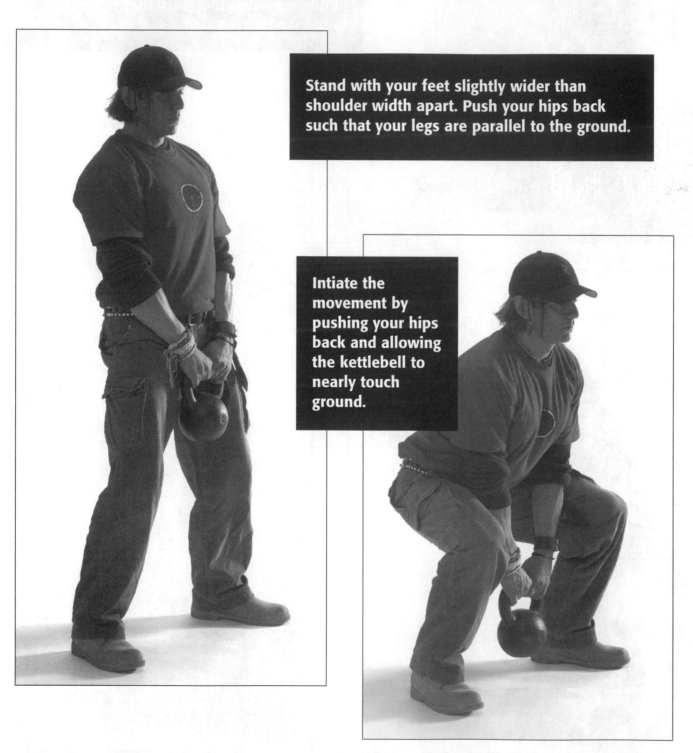

Stand with your feet slightly wider than shoulder width apart. Push your hips back such that your legs are parallel to the ground.

Intiate the movement by pushing your hips back and allowing the kettlebell to nearly touch ground.

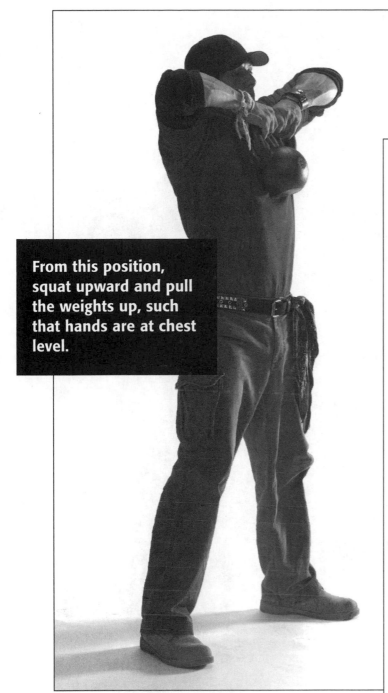

From this position, squat upward and pull the weights up, such that hands are at chest level.

Renegade Squat-Pull on Swiss Ball

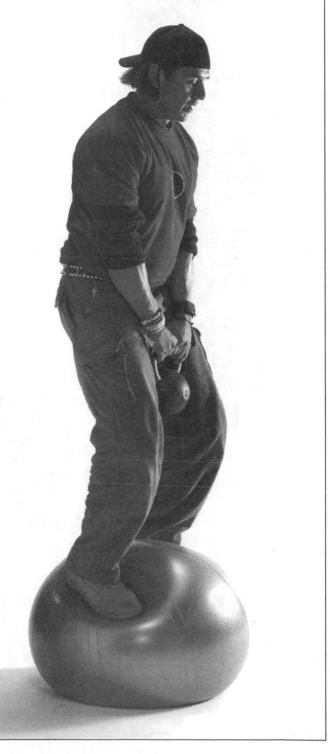

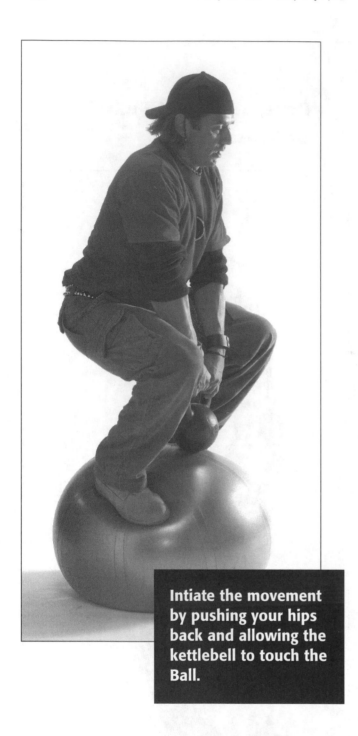

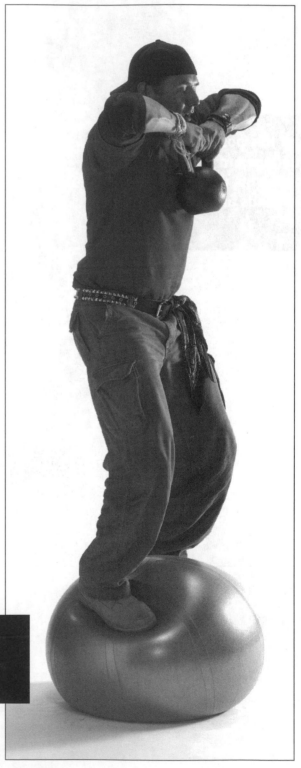

Intiate the movement by pushing your hips back and allowing the kettlebell to touch the Ball.

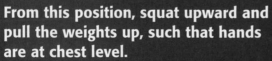

From this position, squat upward and pull the weights up, such that hands are at chest level.

Towel Chins

Drape a towel over the bar, and grab onto the ends. Pull yourself up until your chin clears the bar, and then lower yourself again.

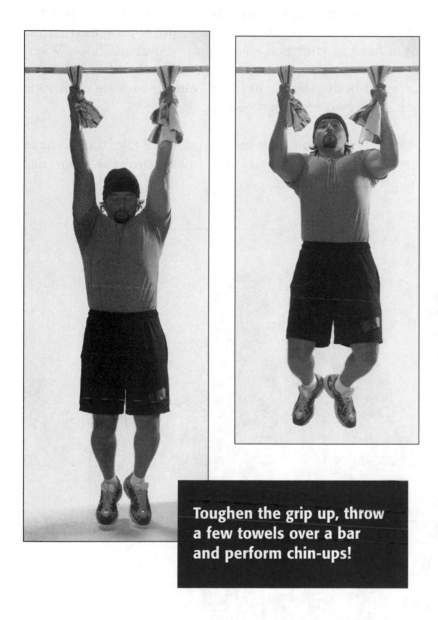

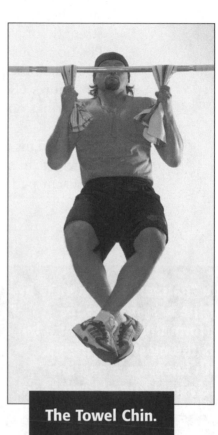

The Towel Chin.

Toughen the grip up, throw a few towels over a bar and perform chin-ups!

Natural Glute/Ham Raise

Begin in a kneeling position, such that the tops of your feet are pressed against the ground. Have a training partner push down on your heels to resist your movement. Keeping the line from your knees to your torso perfectly straight, slowly lean forward and lower your body to the ground. Use the strength of your glute and hamstring muscles to control your movement. Position your hands in front of your body as you move near the floor. When you touch the floor, explosively push yourself up with your hands (as if doing a pushup). Use your upper-body strength to bring yourself back up until your hamstrings and glutes are strong enough to do so.

Notes: This is an incredibly difficult movement, and it will take time to have sufficient ham/glute strength to master it. Also make sure the floor has sufficient padding to protect your knees.

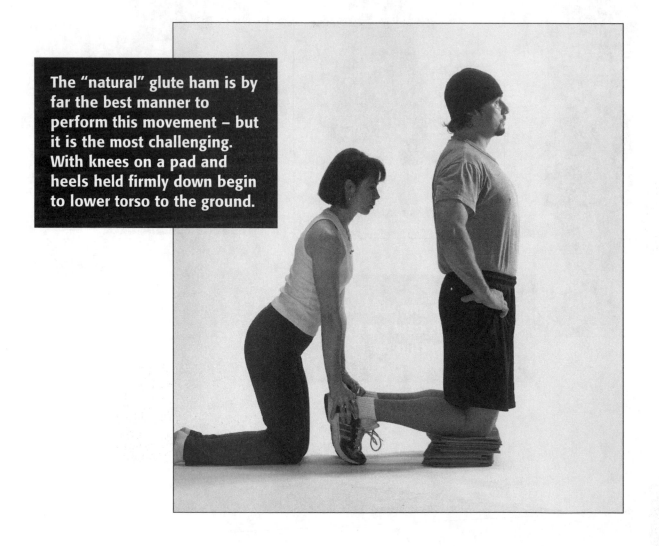

The "natural" glute ham is by far the best manner to perform this movement – but it is the most challenging. With knees on a pad and heels held firmly down begin to lower torso to the ground.

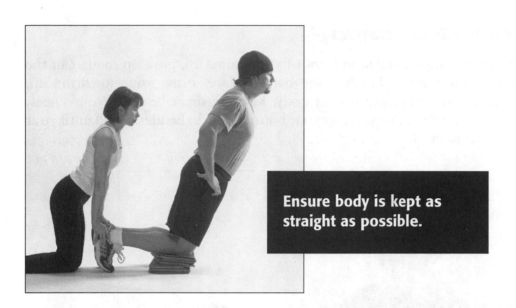

Ensure body is kept as straight as possible.

As hamstrings give out – allow body to come down to push out position and explode upward.

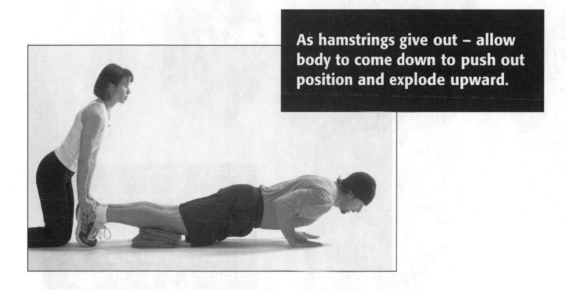

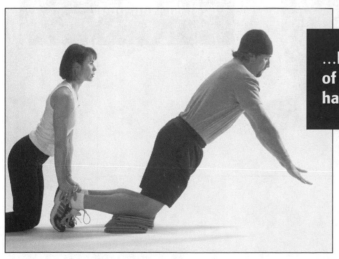

...but with only a slight amount of momentum until your hamstrings can pull yourself up.

Zercher "Good Morning"

With your arms extended in front of you, palms up, position the bar in the crooks of your arms. Holding the bar in place, bring your forearms up, squeezing them tight against your body. Keeping slight bends in your knees, initiate the movement by pushing your buttocks back. Bend forward until your back is at a neutral.

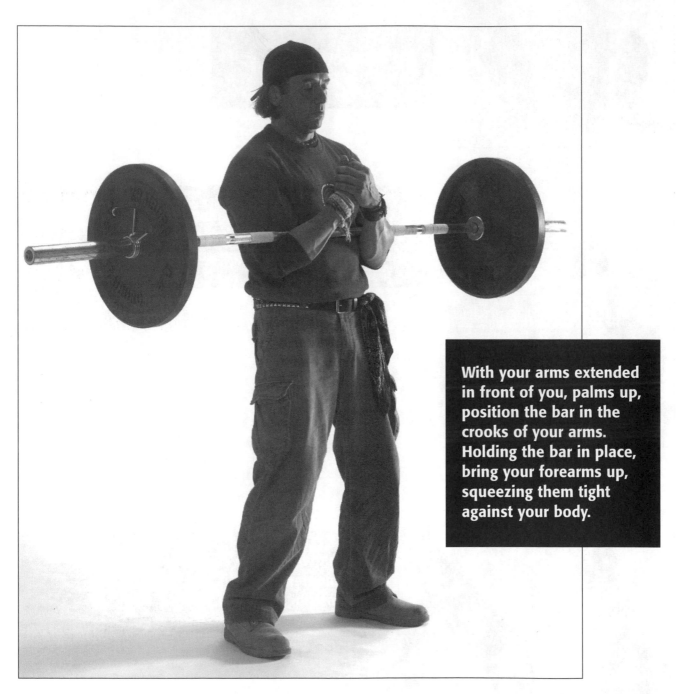

With your arms extended in front of you, palms up, position the bar in the crooks of your arms. Holding the bar in place, bring your forearms up, squeezing them tight against your body.

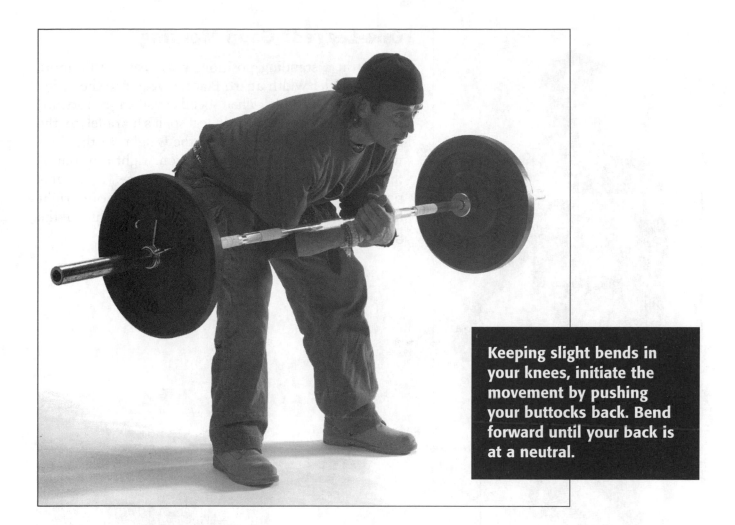

Keeping slight bends in your knees, initiate the movement by pushing your buttocks back. Bend forward until your back is at a neutral.

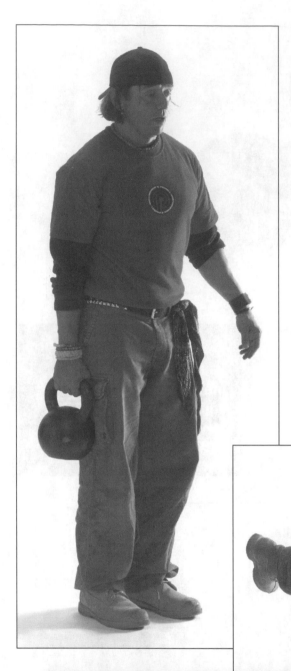

One-Legged "Good Morning"

Begin in a standing position, your feet a little more than shoulder width apart. Place a weight to the inside of your right foot. Then bend over in a forward direction and lift your left leg so it's parallel to the ground but slightly bent. Grab the weight off the floor with your left hand, and stretch your right arm out to the side to help maintain your balance. From this position, stand upright, pulling with your right hamstring as you do so. Lower the weight to the ground, and repeat the entire movement.

Bend over in a forward direction and lift your left leg so it's parallel to the ground but slightly bent. Grab the weight off the floor with your left hand, and stretch your right arm out to the side to help maintain your balance. From this position, stand upright, pulling with your right hamstring as you do so.

Side Press

Begin in a standing position. Hold a dumbbell or kettlebell in one hand, and extend that arm straight out to the side at shoulder height. Put the other hand on your hip, with your arm bent and out to the side. Push the weight above your head while you bend to the opposite side. Then straighten out again.

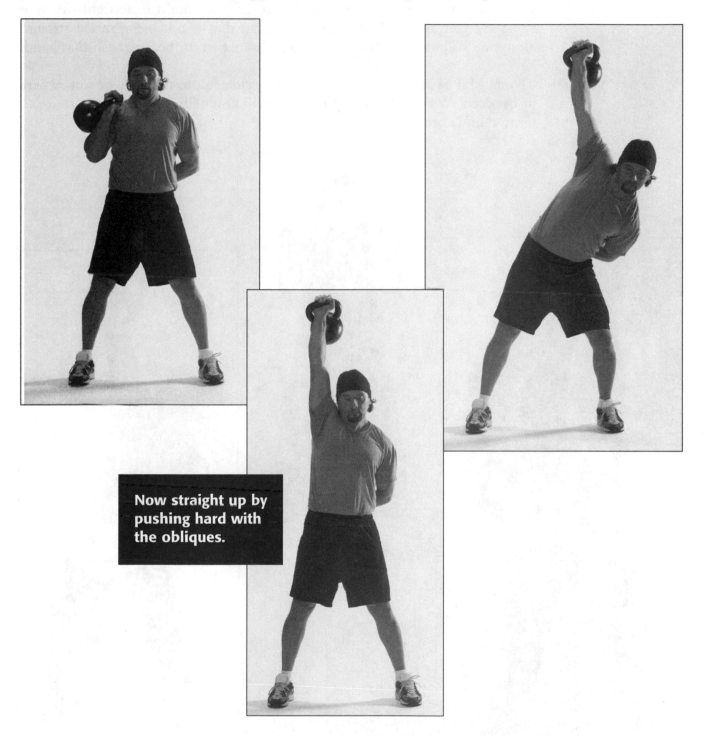

Now straight up by pushing hard with the obliques.

See-Saw Press

Begin in a standing position, your legs slightly more than shoulder width apart. Hold a kettlebell in each hand, your arms down at your sides. Beginning with your right arm, drive the weight straight up as you bend to the left side. Then lower your arm and bend back to an upright position. Next, make the same movements but with your left arm and bending to the right side and back. As you alternate arms, keep the arm that is not being raised straight alongside your body. You should feel resistance from the weight in that hand.

Note: Make sure you bend directly to the side, not to the front or somewhere in between. With continued effort, you will gradually improve your range of motion and core strength.

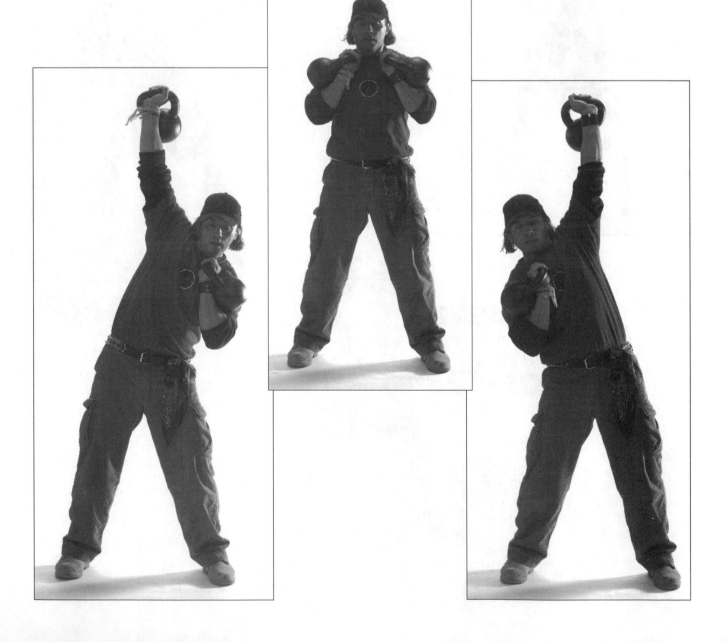

See-Saw Press on Balance Ball

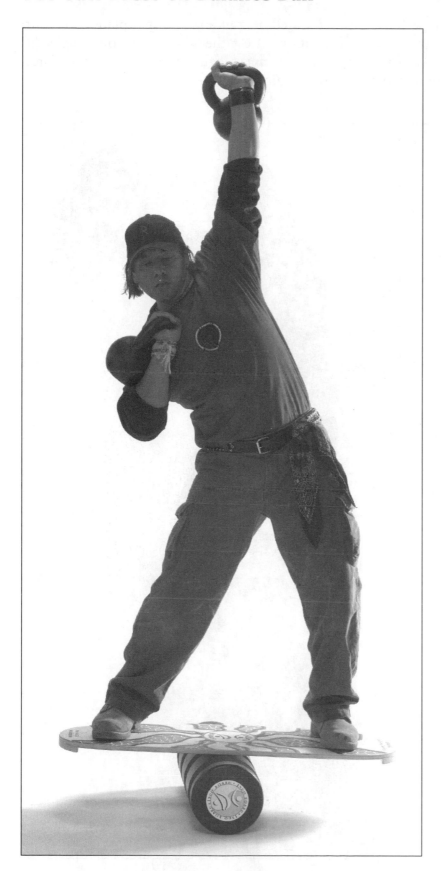

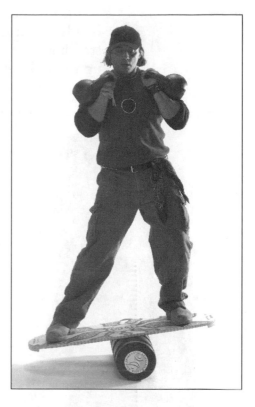

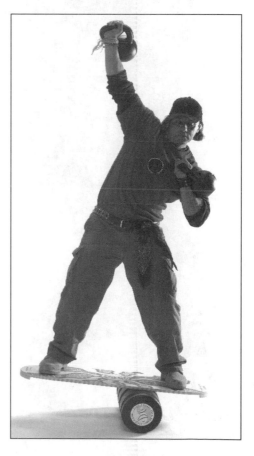

Plate Raise

This lift can be performed either seated or standing. Grasp a plate with your hands at the 3 and 9 o'clock positions. Rest the weight on your thighs (if standing) or your forearms against your inner thighs (if seated). Lift the plates up to eye level and then back down again.

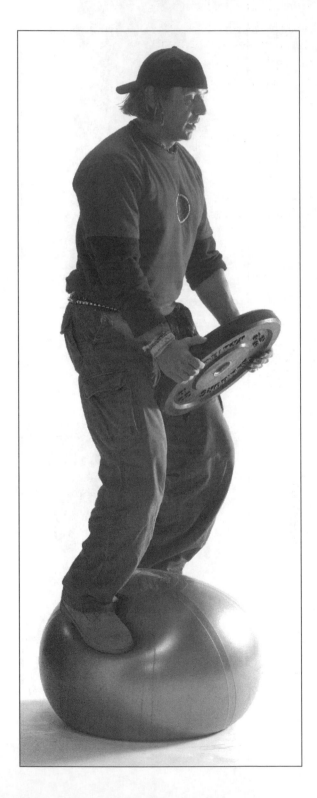
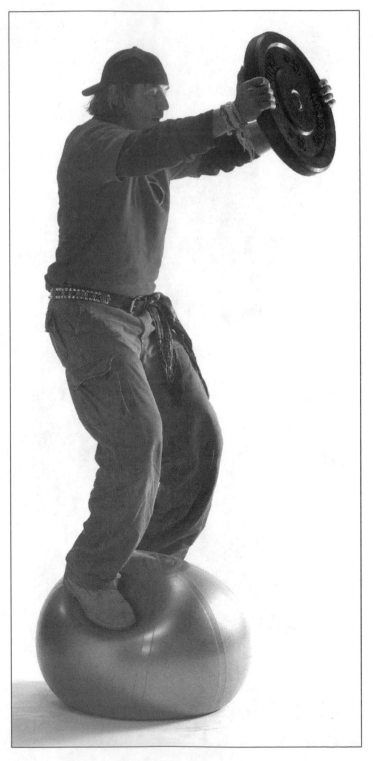

Bradford Press

Begin in a standing position. Rest the bar on the backs of your shoulders in a typical back squat. Using a snatch grip, push the weight off your shoulders and raise it to slightly above head level. Then lower the bar, coming in front of your head and continuing down until the bar touches your chest. Reverse these movements, lifting the bar up and over your head and then down behind your head and onto the backs of you shoulders. This entire sequence counts as one rep.

Note: The width of your grip should vary from set to set to avoid adaptation. I generally start with a grip that's similar in width to the snatch grip and bring it in a few inches each set.

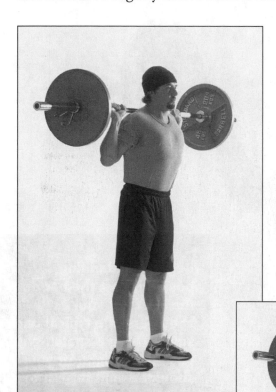

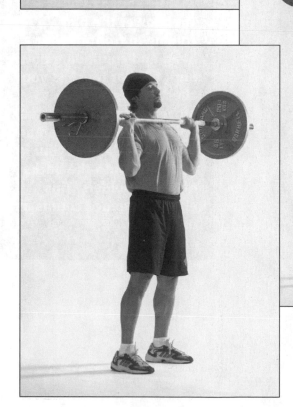

Bradford Press on Balance Board

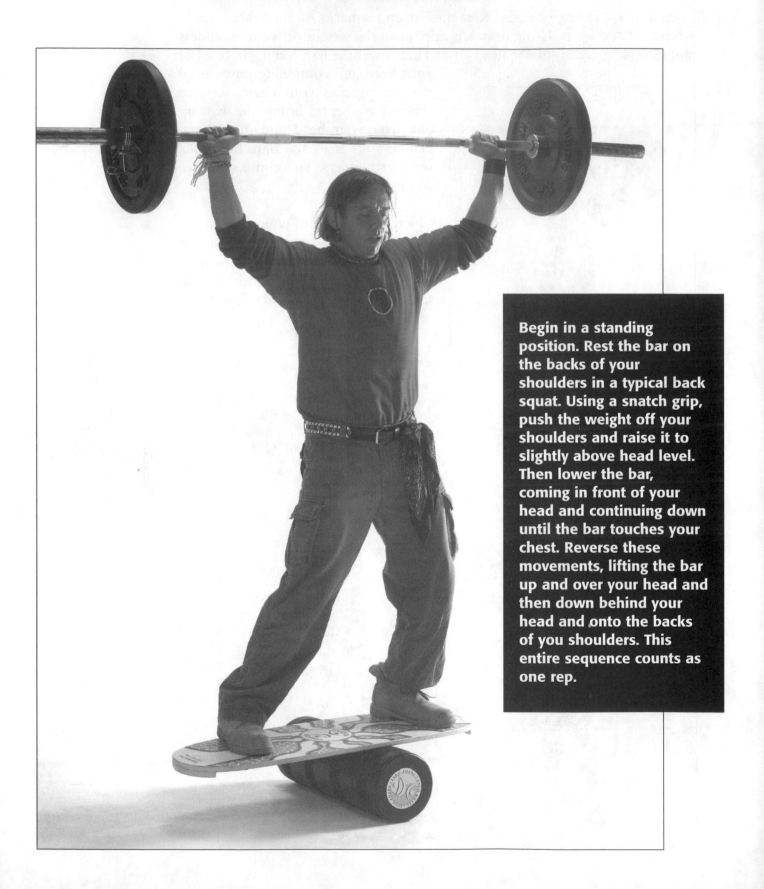

Begin in a standing position. Rest the bar on the backs of your shoulders in a typical back squat. Using a snatch grip, push the weight off your shoulders and raise it to slightly above head level. Then lower the bar, coming in front of your head and continuing down until the bar touches your chest. Reverse these movements, lifting the bar up and over your head and then down behind your head and onto the backs of you shoulders. This entire sequence counts as one rep.

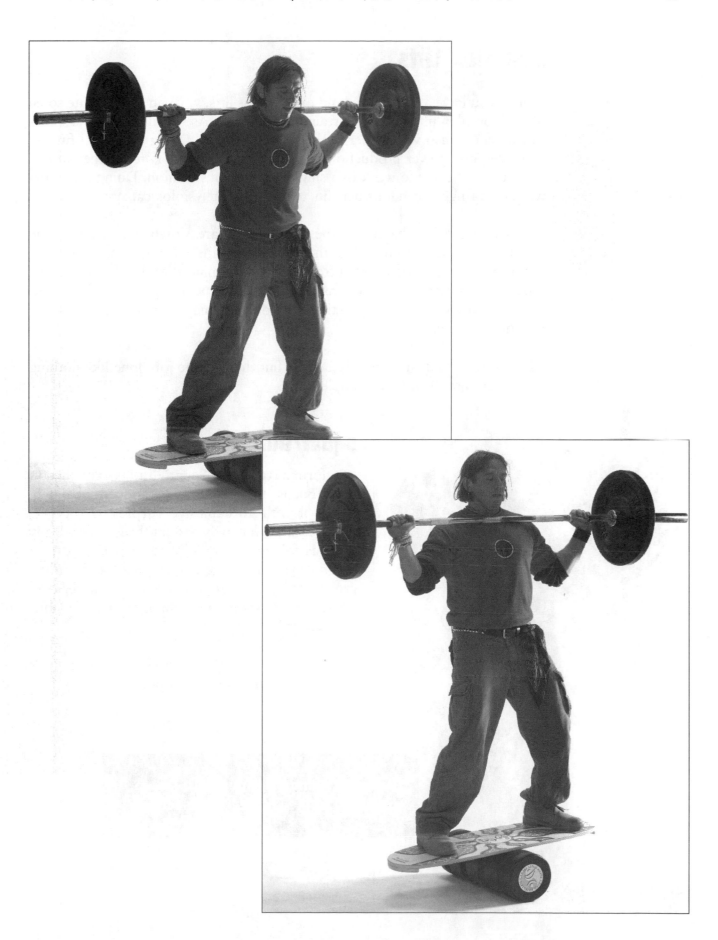

Complex Lifts

Once you have a solid command of the focus lifts, you can incorporate some of the complex lifts into your training programs. As noted earlier, these lifts can be performed with either barbells or kettlebells. Doing them will further enhance your power production and endurance as well as teach the various parts of your body to work in a single, harmonious fashion. Doing these lifts will also bring tremendous benefits to your total physiological system.

As you'll see in Chapter 7, these complexes are slowly written into the training program. And while they provide some of the best and most important elements of strength training, keep in mind that they are advanced lifts. Take care at all times to ensure good technique and postural alignment. In fact, make sure you are practicing good technique before you even start to use the complexes.

The complex lifts are brutally taxing, but they get the job done like nothing else. There are three basic complex lifts:

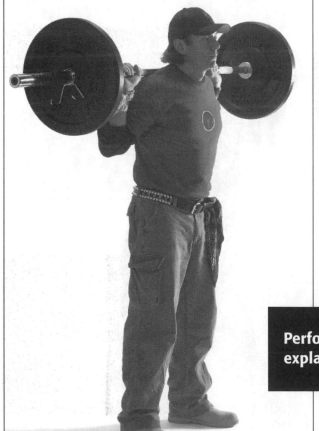

Squat/Burpee

Perform a standard "Squat" lift (as explained in the "Focus Lifts" section), and immediately follow it with 10 explosive burpees. (A burpee, which is also known as a squat thrust, is basically done as follows: From a standing position, drop down to your haunches, place your hands on the ground as in a pushup position, kick your legs out straight behind you, jump out as high as possible, and repeat.)

Note: This is likely the easiest of the complex lifts from a compliance standpoint.

Perform a standard "Squat" lift (as explained in the "Focus Lifts" section)

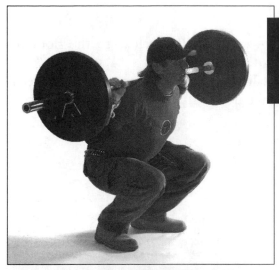

Perform a standard "Squat"...

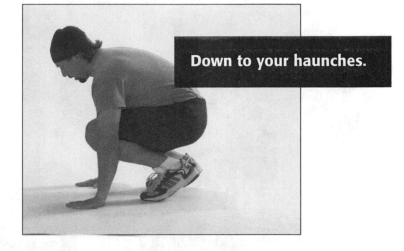

Down to your haunches.

...and immediately follow it with 10 explosive burpees.

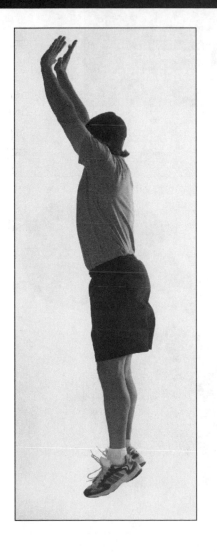

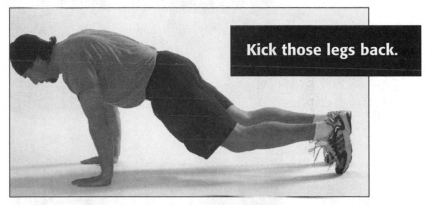

Kick those legs back.

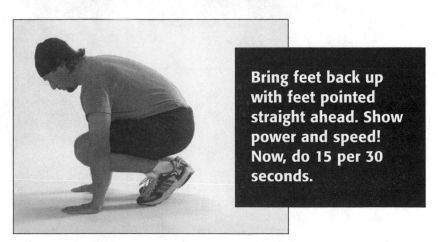

Bring feet back up with feet pointed straight ahead. Show power and speed! Now, do 15 per 30 seconds.

Squat/Push Press

From the standard squat position, lower yourself as close to the floor as possible, and then drive the weight up as you perform a "Push press" (as explained in the "Focus Lifts" section). In performing this complex lift, your intensity level should correspond to that used in performing your maximal "Push press" lift.

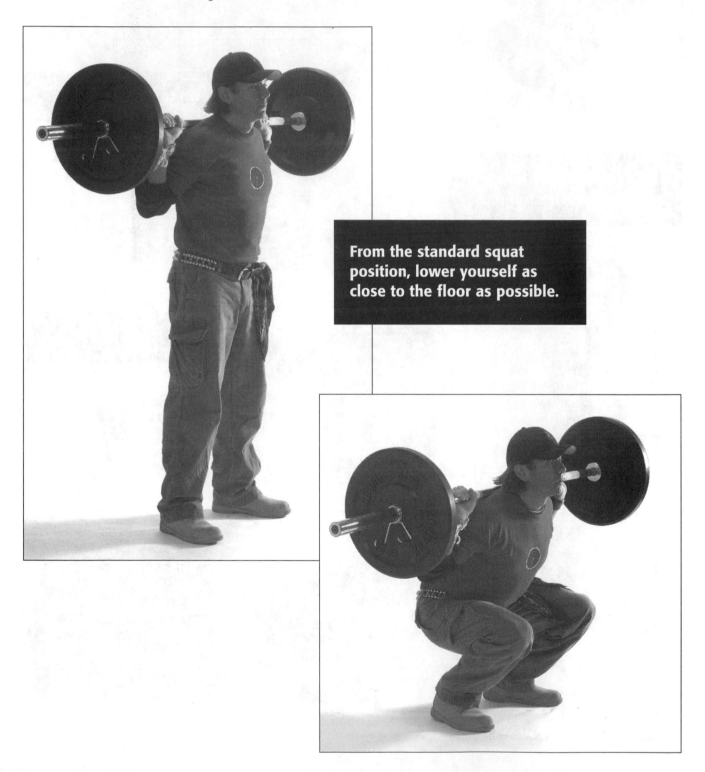

From the standard squat position, lower yourself as close to the floor as possible.

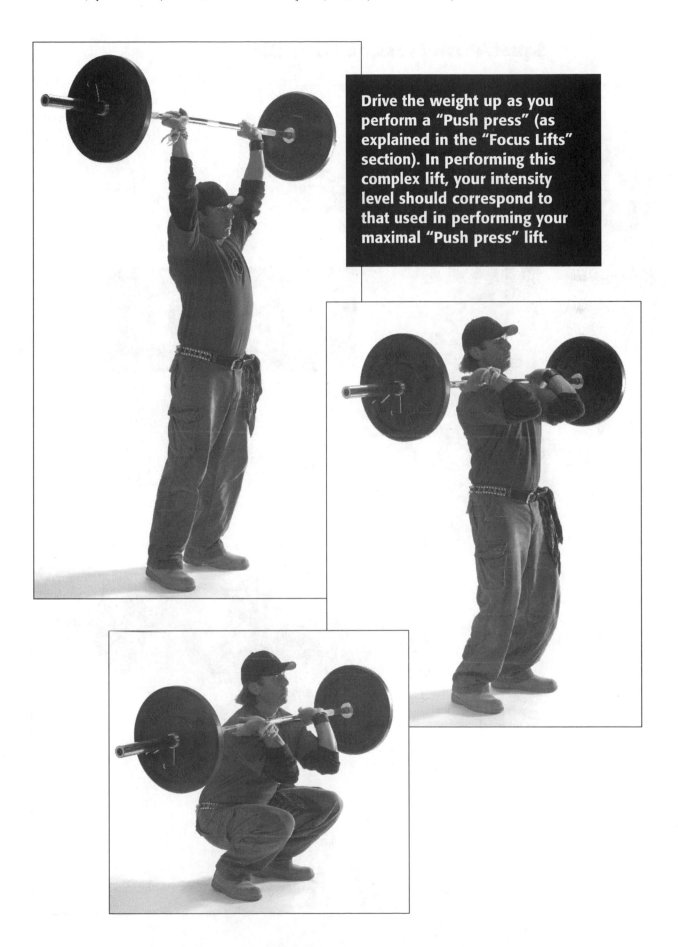

Drive the weight up as you perform a "Push press" (as explained in the "Focus Lifts" section). In performing this complex lift, your intensity level should correspond to that used in performing your maximal "Push press" lift.

Squat/Push Press on Swiss Ball

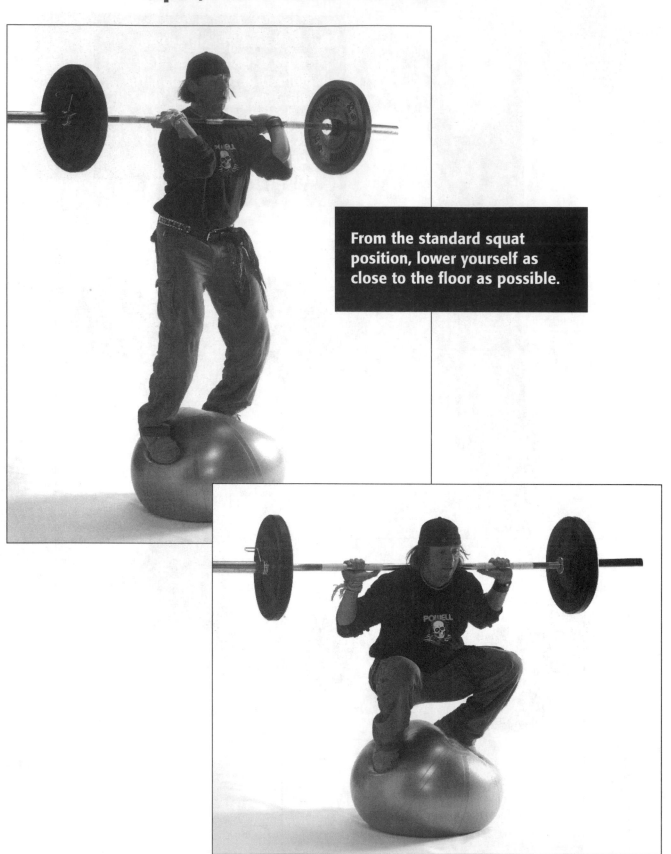

From the standard squat position, lower yourself as close to the floor as possible.

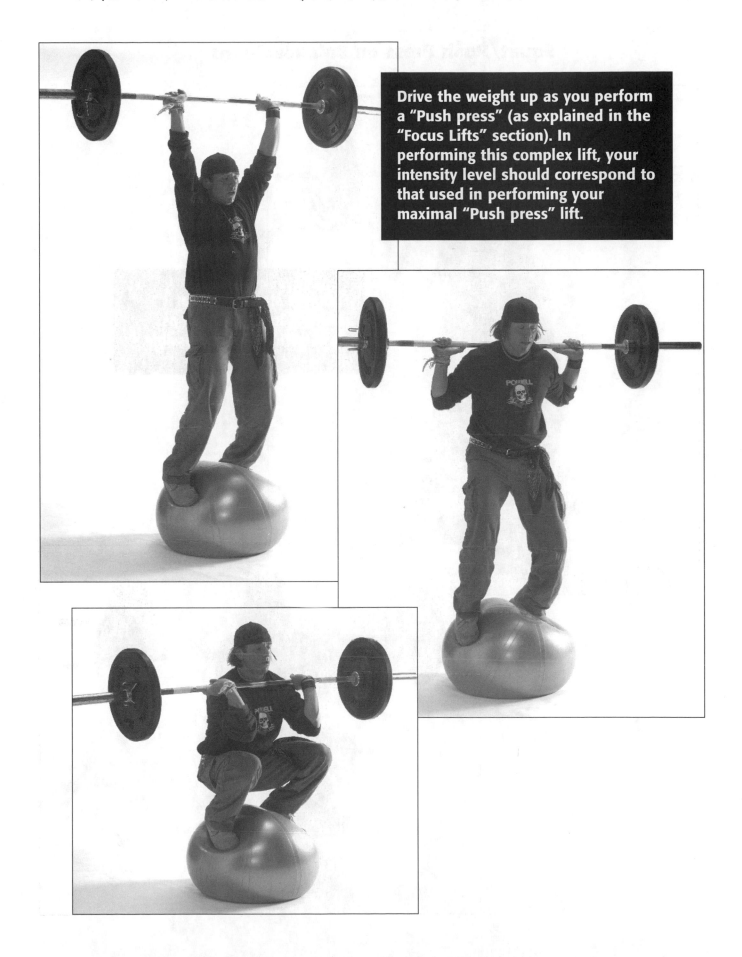

Drive the weight up as you perform a "Push press" (as explained in the "Focus Lifts" section). In performing this complex lift, your intensity level should correspond to that used in performing your maximal "Push press" lift.

Squat/Push Press on Balance B0ard

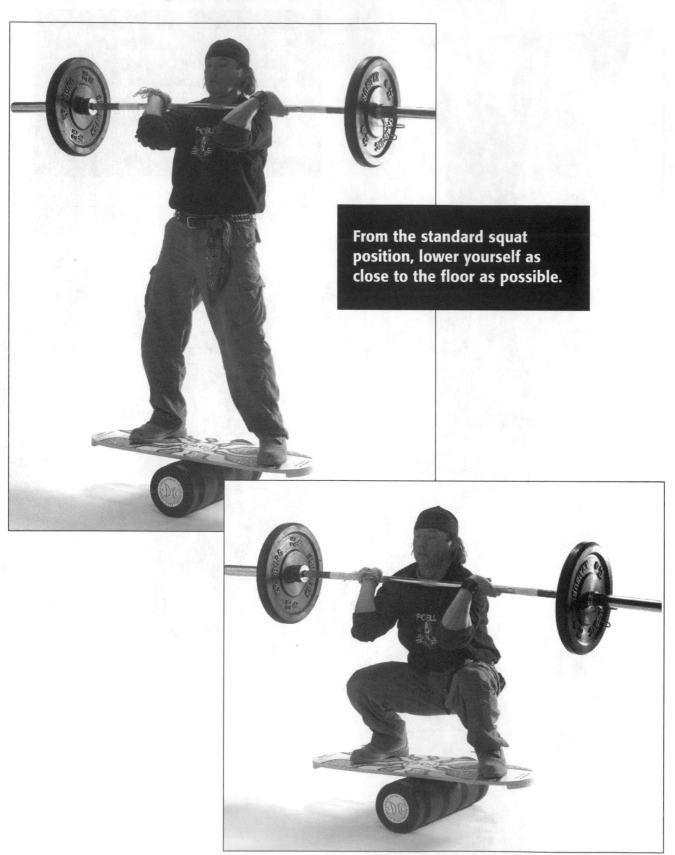

From the standard squat position, lower yourself as close to the floor as possible.

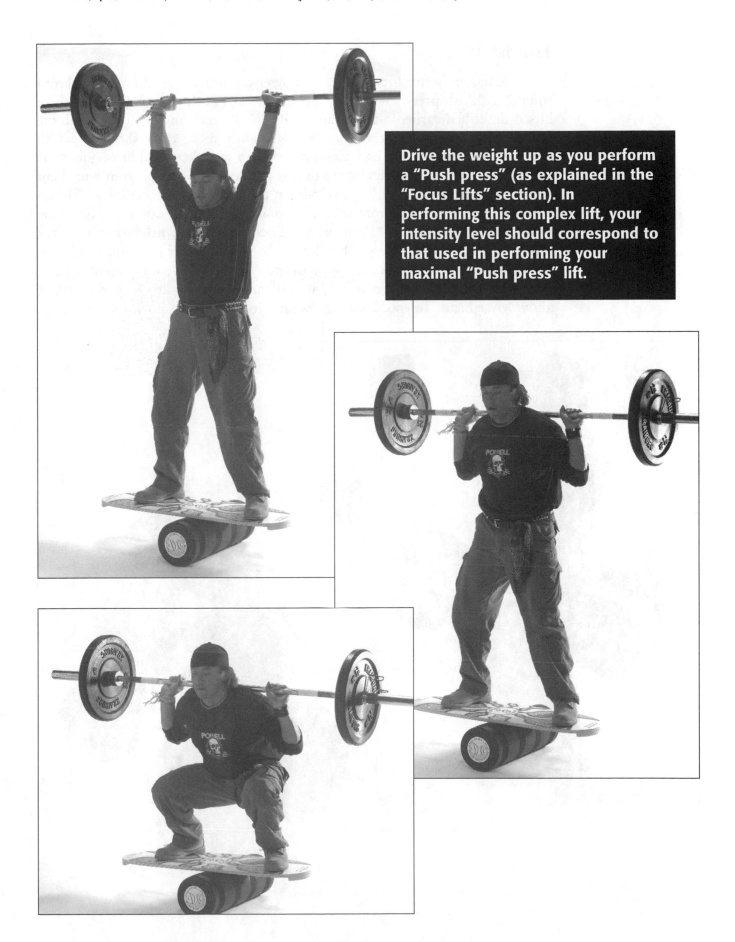

Drive the weight up as you perform a "Push press" (as explained in the "Focus Lifts" section). In performing this complex lift, your intensity level should correspond to that used in performing your maximal "Push press" lift.

The Bear

This is basically five lifts in one: a "Power clean (hang position)," a "Front squat," a "Push press," a "Squat," and another "Push press." (Each of these lifts is described earlier in this chapter.) Begin in a standing position. Grab the bar with an overhand grip, your hands slightly more than shoulder width apart. Keep your head up and your eyes focused straight ahead throughout the total movement. Drop quickly into the proper neutral position, your back bent at about 45 degrees, and then explode up to perform a "Power clean." From there, drop into a full "Front squat," and as you begin to come up, drive the weight up to perform a "Push press." Lock your arms, holding the weight above your head, and pause. Then lower the weight to behind your head, and drop into a "Squat." From the base of the "Squat," drive the weight up and perform another "Push press." Again, at the top of the lift, lock the weight above your head. To end, lower the weight to the starting position.

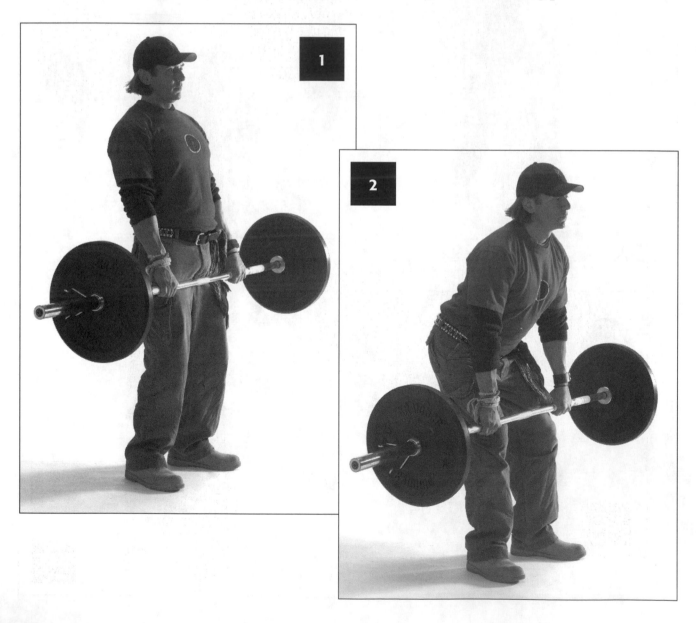

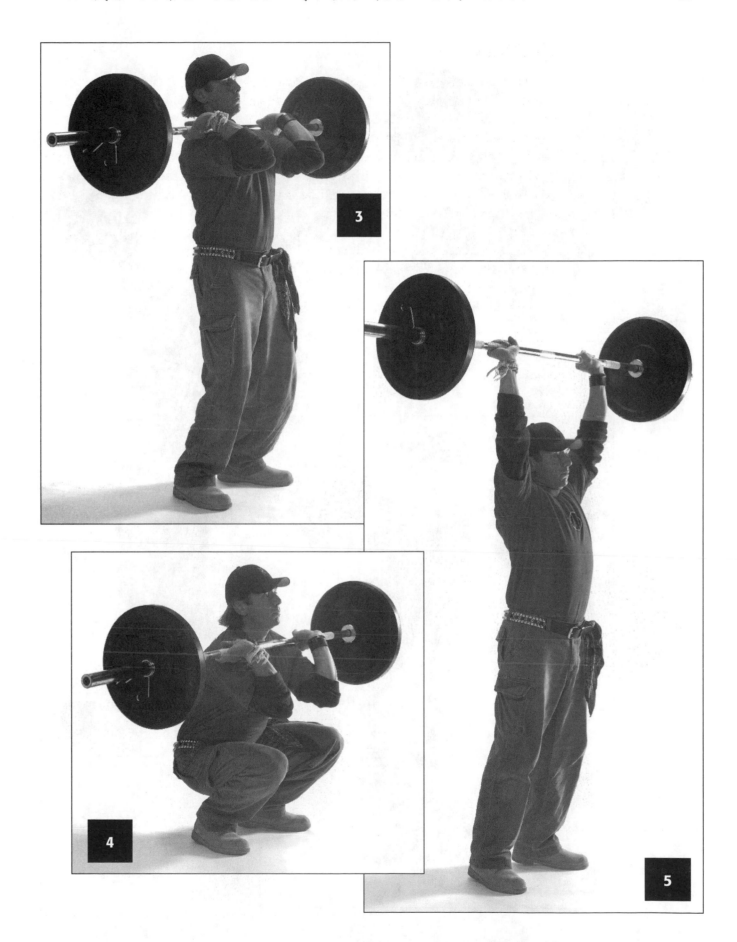

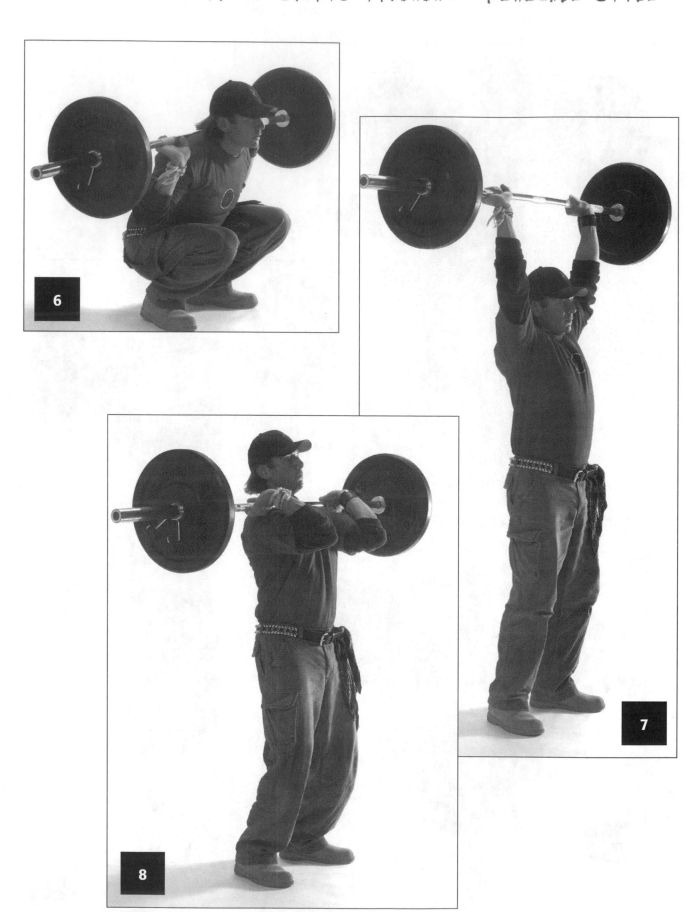

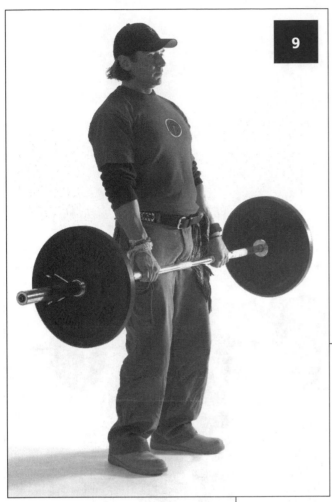

The Bear on Swiss Ball

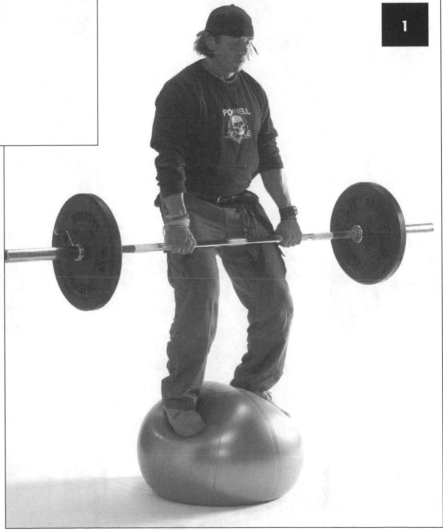

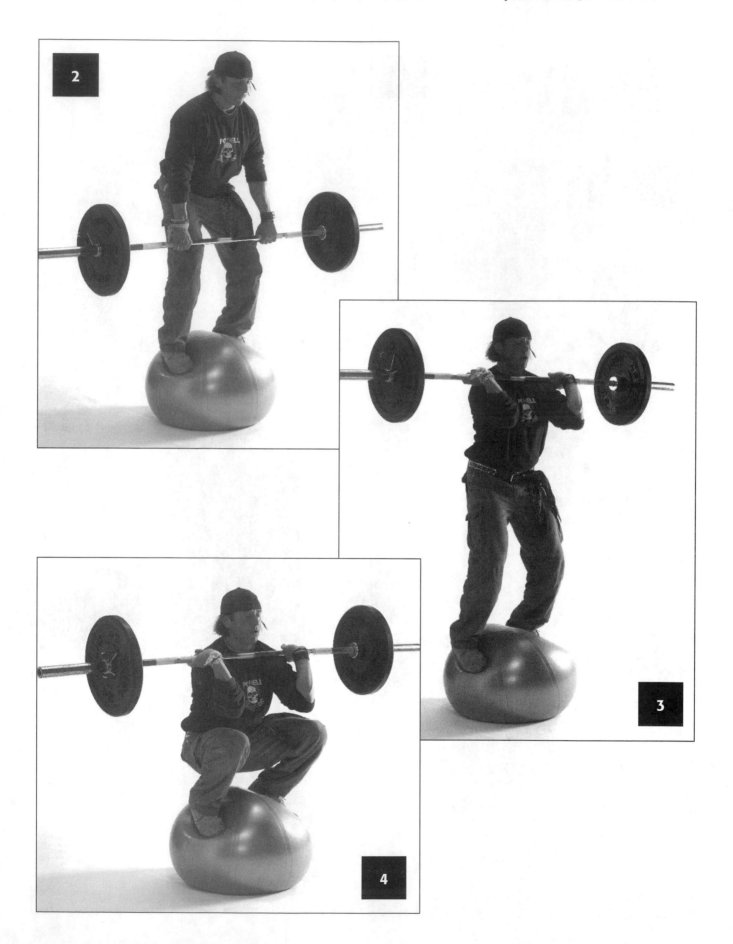

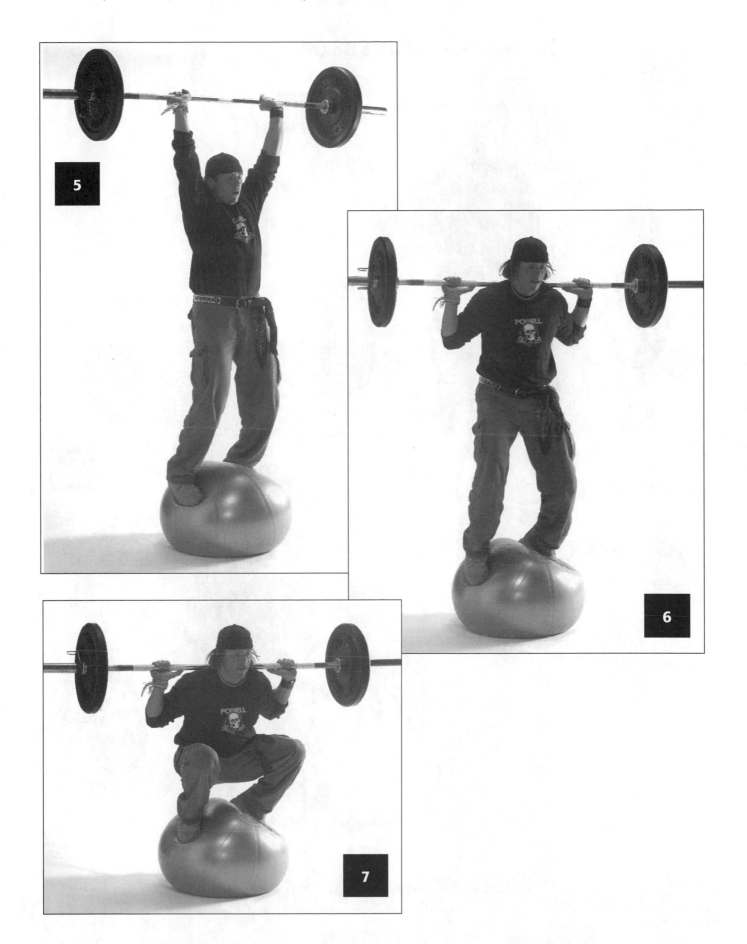

The Bear on Balance Board

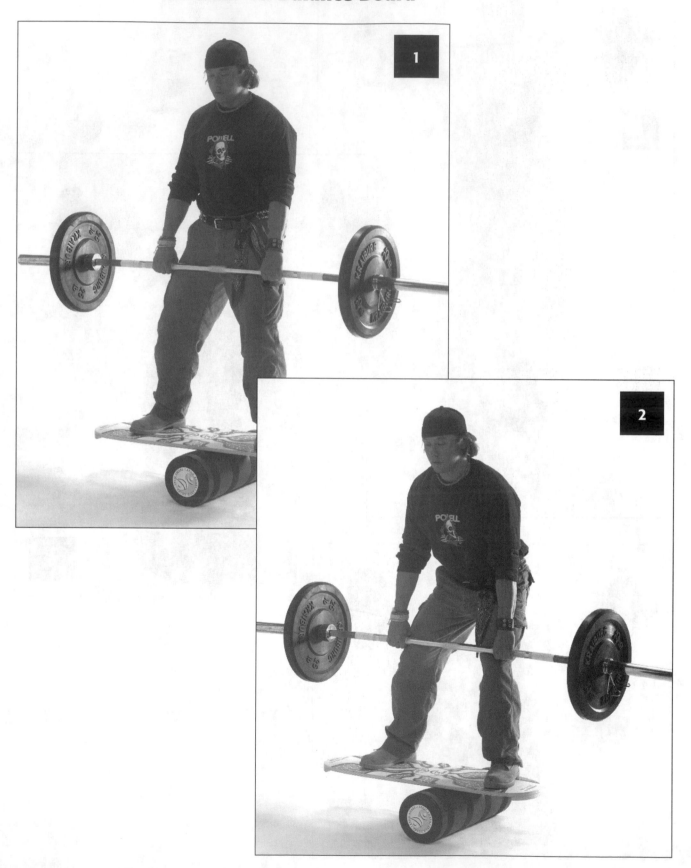

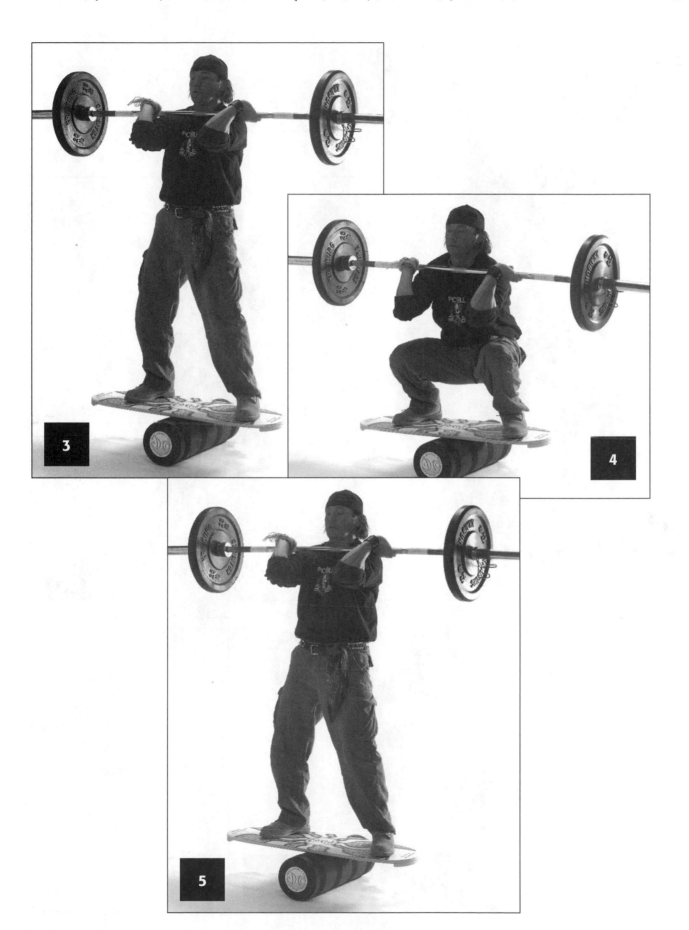

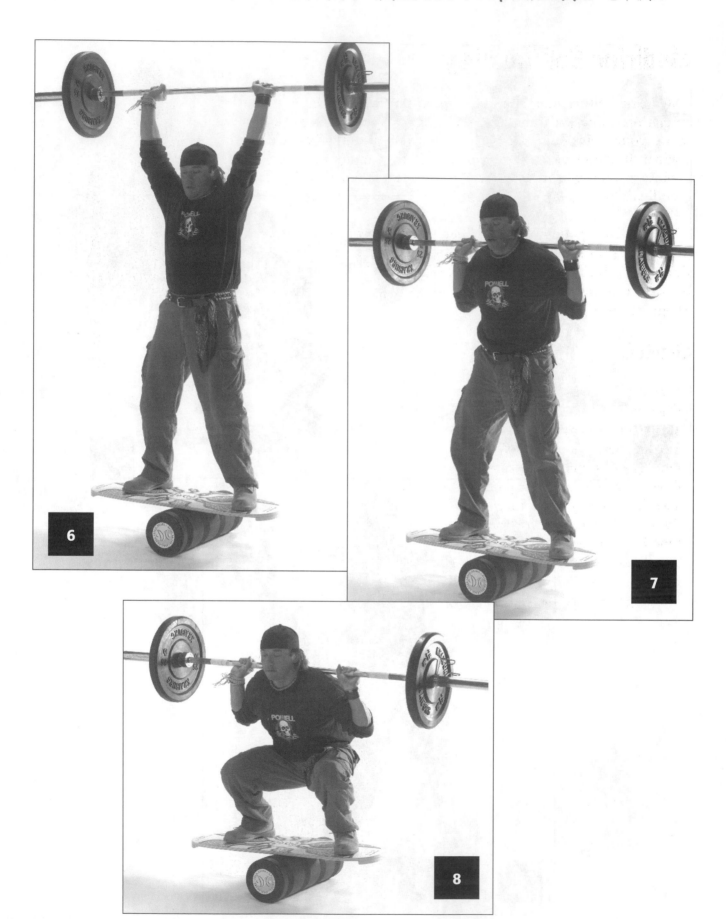

Medicine Ball Training

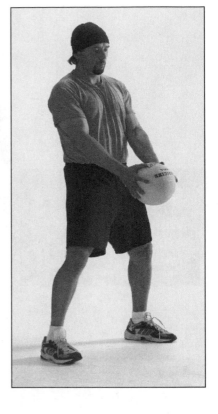

Medicine ball training is another important part of the Renegade strength-training program. The purpose of "med" ball work is to make your neuromuscular system move with total balance and control. It complements the balance of your training by developing explosive power, core stability, proprioception, and eye/hand coordination.

The med ball training uses a basic circuit, in which all drills are performed while moving comfortably on the balance board. (See Chapter 3, the section on "Balance Training," for more on this board.) You will make 50 throws in each circuit using a 3 to 5 kilogram (max.) ball.

Circuit 1

Perform 5 throws per motion; move in continuous fashion
Chest pass
Step-in chest pass (right forward)
Step-in chest pass (left forward)
One-hand twisting chest pass (right forward)
One-hand twisting chest pass (left forward)
Two-hand swing (right forward)
Two-hand swing (left forward)
One-hand swing (right forward)
One-hand swing (left forward)
Overhead pass
Walking overhead pass (right forward)

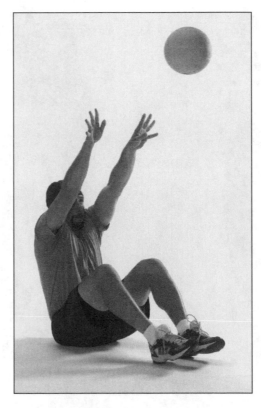

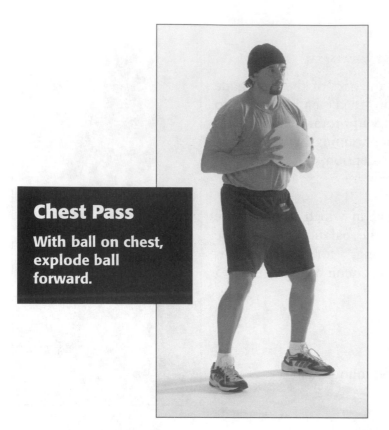

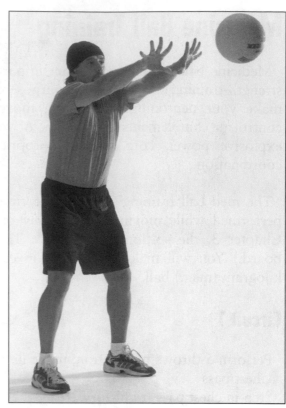

Chest Pass

With ball on chest, explode ball forward.

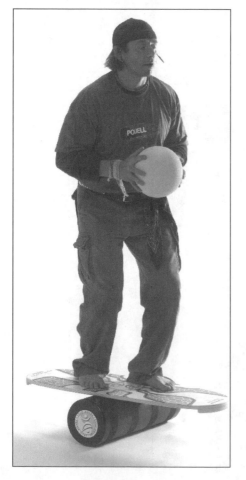

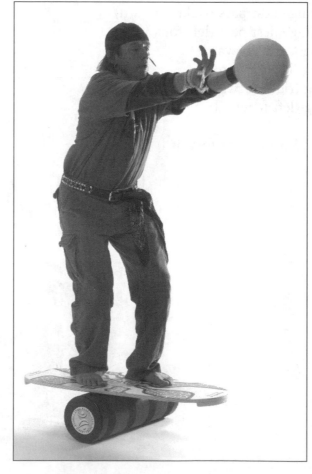

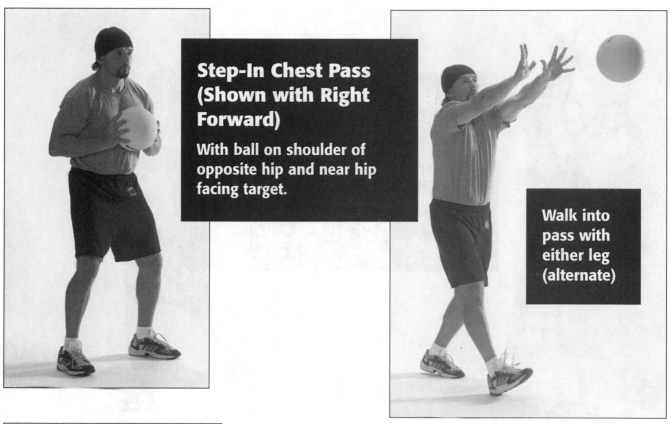

Step-In Chest Pass (Shown with Right Forward)

With ball on shoulder of opposite hip and near hip facing target.

Walk into pass with either leg (alternate)

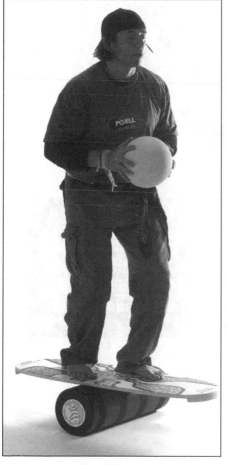

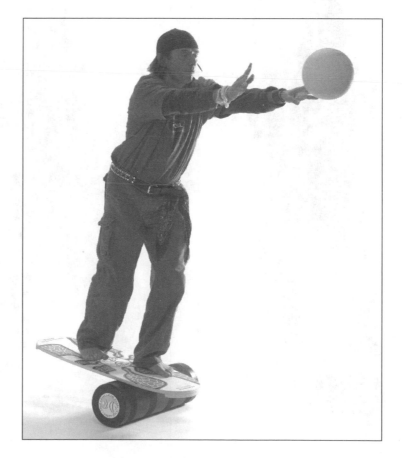

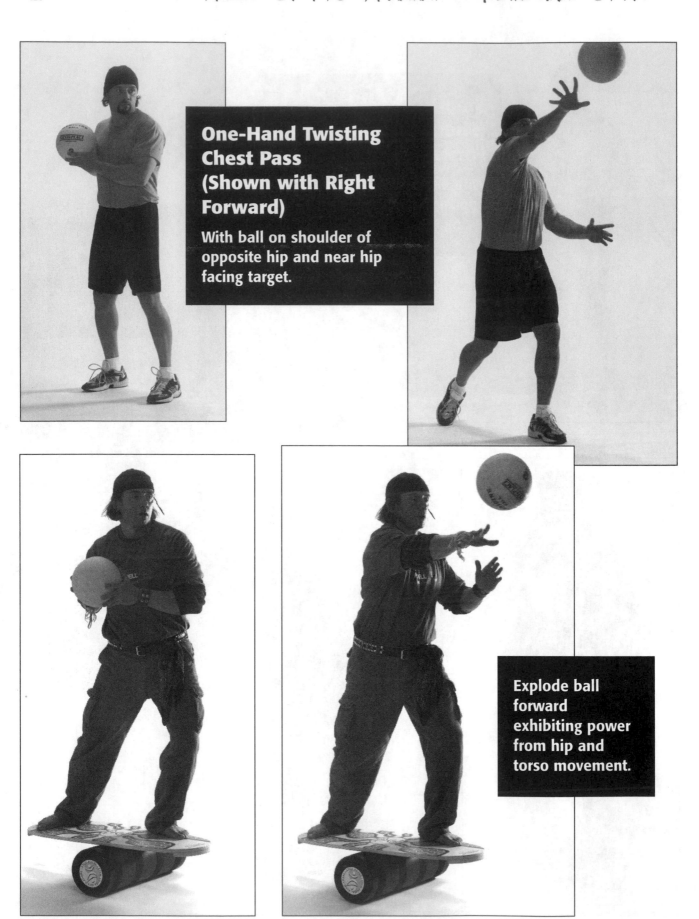

One-Hand Twisting Chest Pass (Shown with Right Forward)

With ball on shoulder of opposite hip and near hip facing target.

Explode ball forward exhibiting power from hip and torso movement.

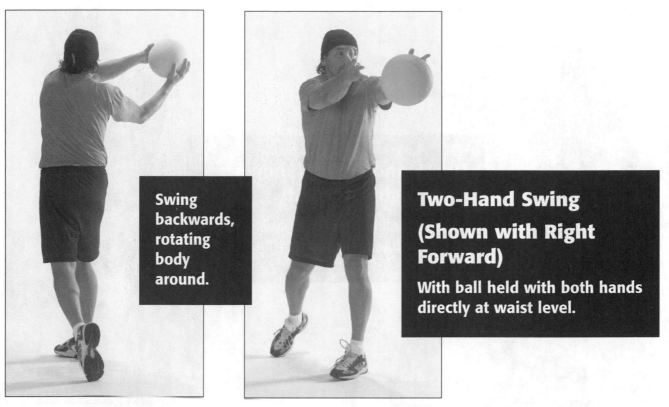

Swing backwards, rotating body around.

Two-Hand Swing (Shown with Right Forward)

With ball held with both hands directly at waist level.

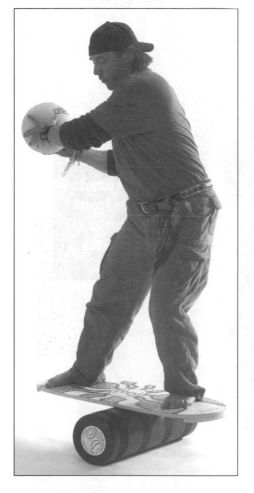

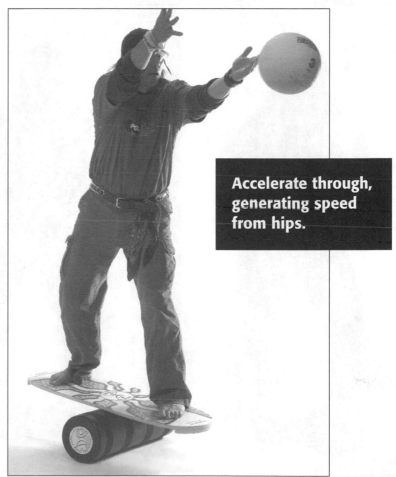

Accelerate through, generating speed from hips.

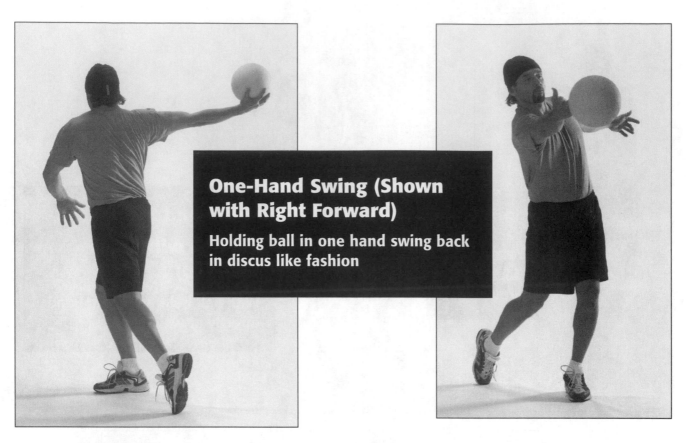

One-Hand Swing (Shown with Right Forward)

Holding ball in one hand swing back in discus like fashion

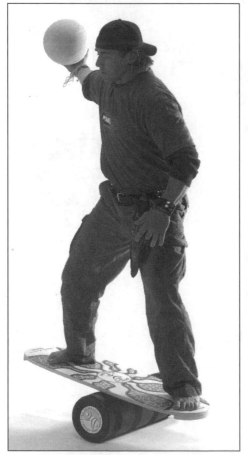

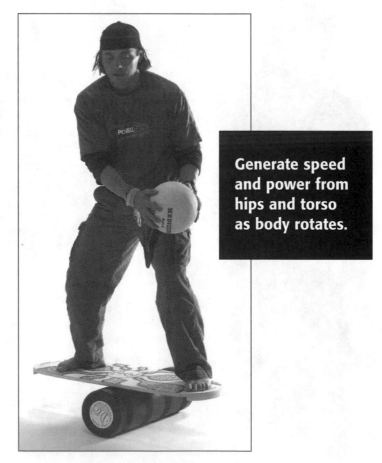

Generate speed and power from hips and torso as body rotates.

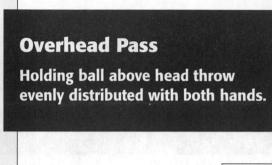

Overhead Pass

Holding ball above head throw evenly distributed with both hands.

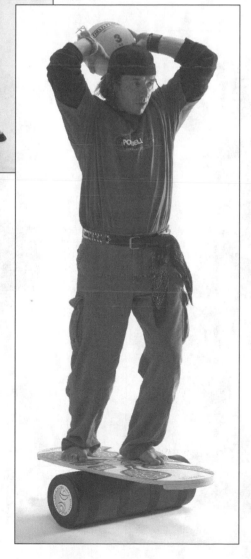

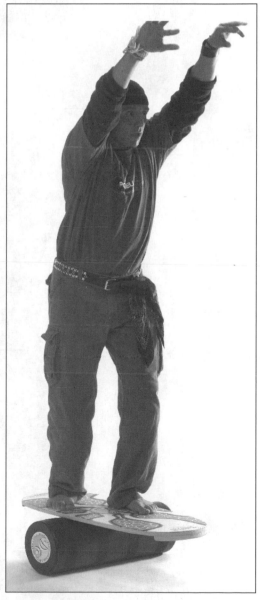

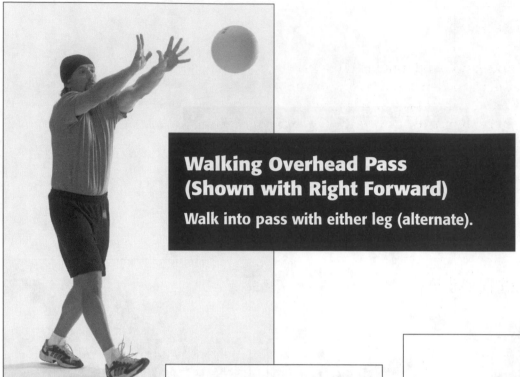

Walking Overhead Pass (Shown with Right Forward)

Walk into pass with either leg (alternate).

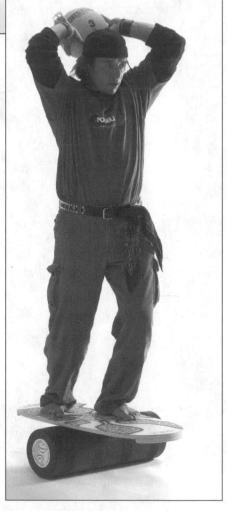

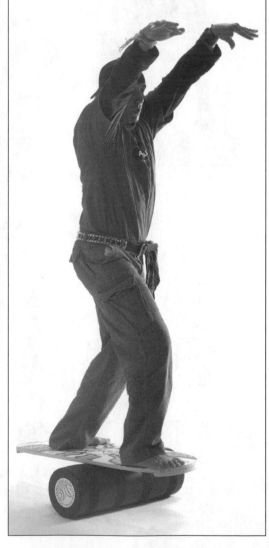

Abdominal Training

Don't think that because abdominal training is the last topic addressed in this chapter on strength development that it is not important or is less important than anything else. Actually, you've been working your abdominal carriage in a many ways throughout Renegade training. The abdominal carriage is involved in all aspects of athletic activity, as it is the center of all movement.

Nonetheless, work your abdominal section even more by doing the following exercises using the set and rep protocols found in the training program in Chapter 7.

Abdominal Exercises

Leg Raise/Pike

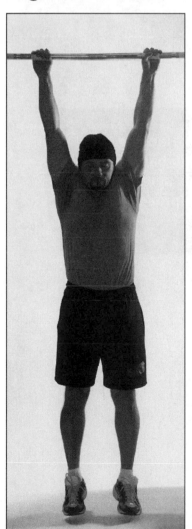

Hang by your arms from a high pullup bar. Keeping your legs and your back straight, raise your legs up until they touch the bar. Lower your legs and repeat the entire movement.

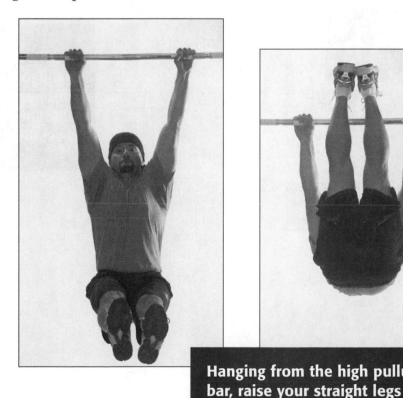

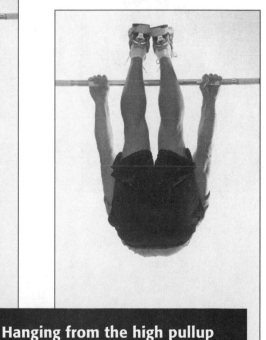

Hanging from the high pullup bar, raise your straight legs upward to touch bar.

Leg Raise/Tuck

Hang by your arms from a high pullup bar. Keeping your back straight but bending your legs at the knees, raise your knees up to your chest. Lower your legs and repeat the entire movement.

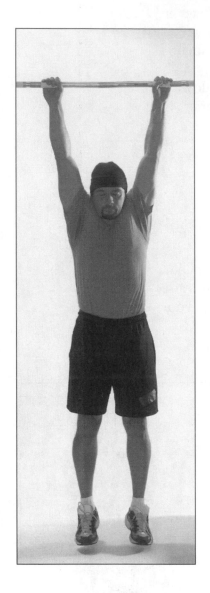

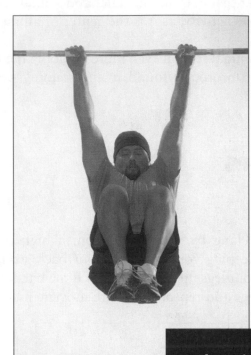

Tuck Position: Hanging from the high pullup bar, raise your bent legs upward until your knees approach your chest area.

Plank

Lay on the ground, positioning yourself to do a pushup. Raise your body using your forearms, and support it in this raised position for 30 seconds. Lower your body and repeat. Be sure to keep your neck, back, and legs straight (hence, the name of this exercise).

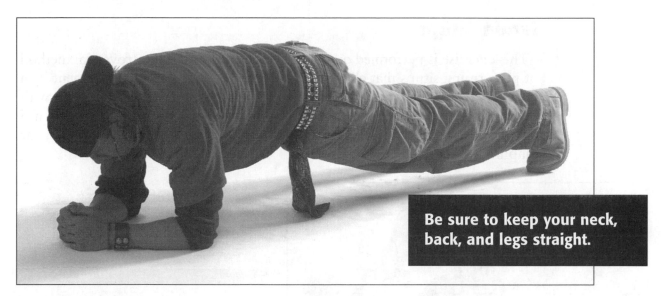

Be sure to keep your neck, back, and legs straight.

Side Plank

Lay on the ground on your right (or left) side. Raise your body using your right (or left) forearm, and support it in this raised position for 30 seconds. Lower your body and repeat. Be sure to keep your neck, back, and legs straight (hence, the name of this exercise).

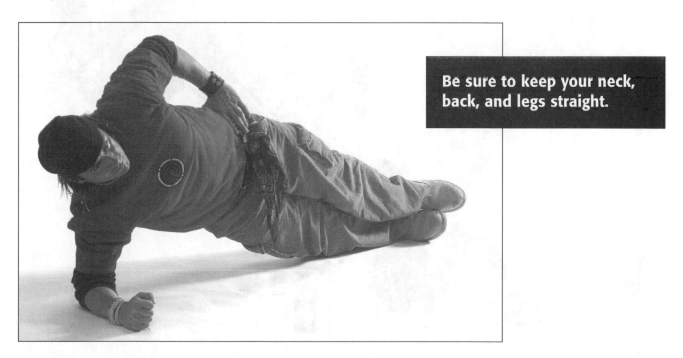

Be sure to keep your neck, back, and legs straight.

Horse Pose (Not Shown)

Sit on all fours, hands and knees. Extend one arm directly forward parallel to the ground while extending opposite leg back parallel to the ground as well. Hold for 30 seconds and change arm / leg position.

Janda Situps

This exercise is performed on the "Pavelizer II." This is controversial method of performing situps that eliminates your hip flexors from the movement by a process called *irradiation*. To perform the exercise, maintain heel contact with the ground and squeeze your glutes and hams tight. Ascend slowly (on a 5 count), squeezing your abdominals tight and slowly releasing air from your diaphragm.

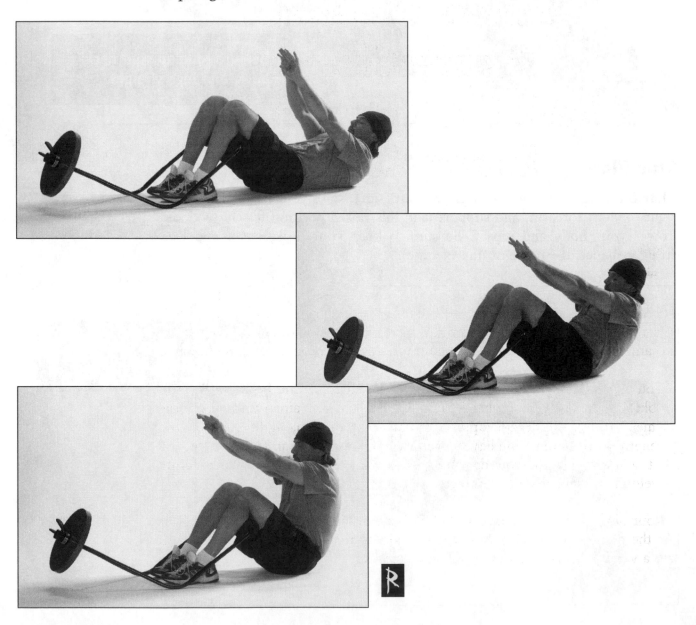

Chapter Six

General Physical Preparation— A Basic Battleplan for The Xtreme Athlete

The overriding philosophy of Renegade Training is that there is a pathway to greatness that, if followed, will lead an athlete toward his or her utmost success. All too often, athletes fail because they don't have a plan that spells out the requirements of the sport and how to go about achieving them. And no amount of hard work will make up for a lack of purpose and planning.

You started along your own pathway to greatness at the beginning of this book, and as you've completed each chapter, you've trained in the essential elements of the Renegade approach: range of motion, agility, speed, and strength. At this point, you have a solid base of knowledge and experience, and that will provide the foundation for the work that remains. Your future development depends on it, in fact!

Your next goal is to achieve a level of General Physical Preparation, or GPP. As the name implies, GPP is a type of training that delicately balances work for a variety of physical development concerns:

- To enhance motor skills
- To train for specific movement patterns that fit sport-specific patterns
- To increase work threshold and, in turn, increase the level of fitness and sport preparation
- To promote active physical recovery
- To promote psychological regeneration for strenuous training
- To provide a transition to Specialized Physical Preparation (SPP) (which is the focus of Chapter 7)

GPP training will also have a positive impact on your mind. As you are able to accomplish these tasks on a regular basis, you will gain confidence and realize that taking a relentless "never say die" approach has brought you tremendous rewards, whether that means you can race down the hill faster, get more air, or accomplish another trick .And as an X-athlete, you need as much of that mindset as you can get!

GPP Exercises

The specific activities you will perform in GPP are extremely diverse and virtually limitless, but in order for them to be effective, you must complete them in precise combinations. You will do an assortment of weighted and nonweighted exercises on a daily basis for a period of time and according to a wave pattern of varying intensities.

Here are some sample patterns of nonweighted GPP exercises. Do each for 30 seconds, and then move on to the next one. Move continuously—without stopping!

Sequence A
- Jumping jacks
- Shuffle splits
- Burpees
- Mountain climbers

Sequence B
- Jumping jacks
- Shuffle splits
- Vertical jumps
- Slalom side-to-side hops

Jumping Jacks

Perform with arms relatively straight and touch at top.

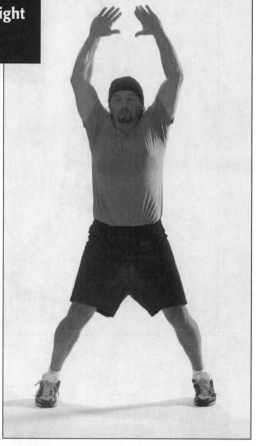

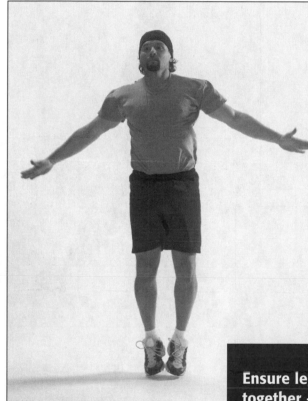

Ensure legs spread wide and come together – perform with discipline and show pride!

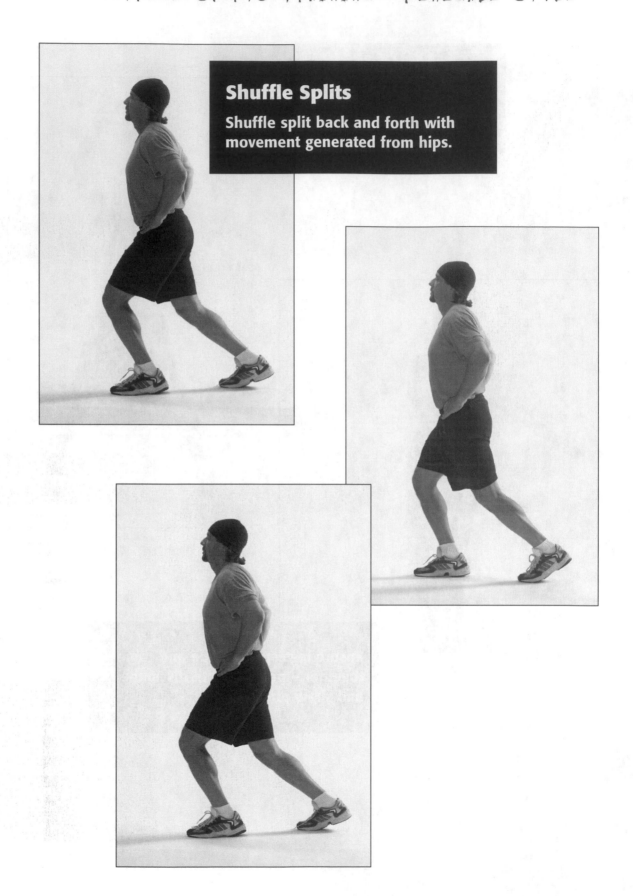

Shuffle Splits

Shuffle split back and forth with movement generated from hips.

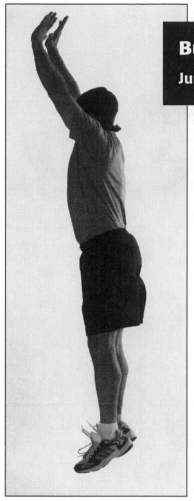

Burpees

Jump up high with arms outstretched.

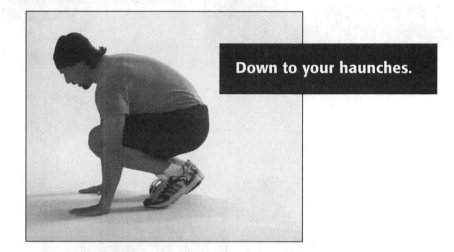

Down to your haunches.

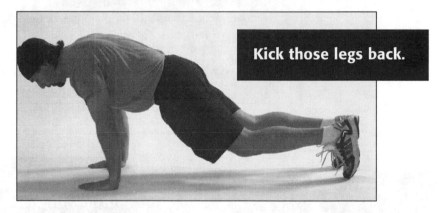

Kick those legs back.

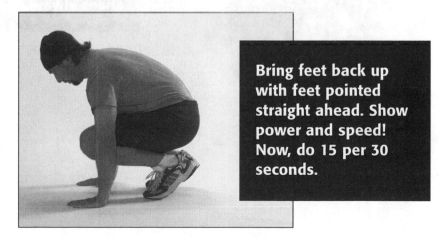

Bring feet back up with feet pointed straight ahead. Show power and speed! Now, do 15 per 30 seconds.

Mountain Climbers

From pushup type position, with one knee up near elbow and other outstretched.

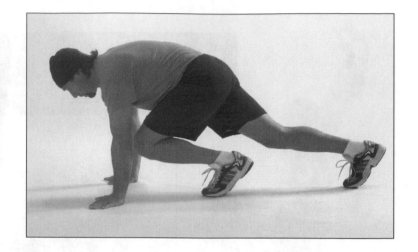

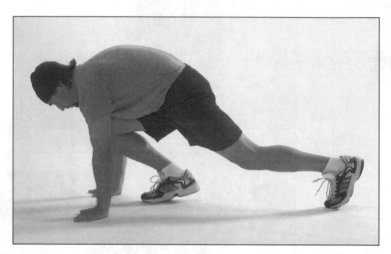

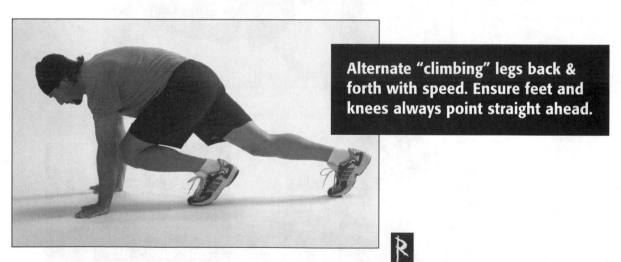

Alternate "climbing" legs back & forth with speed. Ensure feet and knees always point straight ahead.

Chapter Seven

The Renegade Program for Xtreme Xcellence—Putting It All Together

By this time you have reached this chapter, you have done a lot of basic training in a wide range of areas. Now, it's time to put everything together in the most comprehensive training program available, *Renegade style*.

Renegade programs are developed with precise detail with a long term plan in which work is done in an incremental pattern. Programs are developed such that each successive body of work builds upon the prior one, thus building a foundation for future excellence. Each year of training is known as training "Phase" with precise goals and motives. Within each year of training contains training "Levels", periods that last 6 to 8 weeks in duration, that equally possess specific goals and agenda. Quite obviously one of the most challenging and difficult elements to training is getting started on the right path.

Never before published in the public forum, the following is the first Phase of training, Level 1, a 5-day-a-week, 6-week program. Spelled out in precise step-by-step detail over the next few pages it will get you started on your first Xtreme Renegade Training cycle. Remember, this work is neither for the weak or soft of heart but if you want success – this will get you there! and remember "never say die".

—Week One—

Week One • Day One • Sections ABC

Section A	Activity	%E	#S	#R	Notes
Mobility Work	Tumbling		3		
	Dynamic hurdles:				3 set x 5 hurdles
	• Right knee over		3	5	
	• Left knee over		3	5	
	• Down center		3	5	
	Rope routine				
Sprints	Sequence A				
GPP	Sequence A		4		

Section B	Activity	%E	#S	#R	Notes
Quasi SPP	Balance Board				continuous motion
	Squats				30 seconds
	Ollie's		5	5	
	Shuv-its		5	5	
	Cut Back				30 seconds
	Surf - Only				
	Pop-Up		5		
	Hang 10's				30 seconds
	BoardWalks				30 seconds
	Pipeline				30 seconds
	Swiss Ball				
	Ball Dribbles				15 seconds
	Squats				30 seconds
	Back & Forth				30 seconds
	Outside Edge Roll				30 seconds
	Repeat above sequence for 3 sets				

Section C	Activity	%E	#S	#R	Notes
None					

Key code: % E: percent of effort, # S: number of sets, # R: number of reps

Week One • Day One • Sections DE

Section D	Activity	%E	#S	#R	Notes
	Iron Cross	30	2	15	Rest is 60 seconds between sets
	Kettlebell Swings	30	2	15	
	Renegade Squat/Pull	30	2	15	
	1 hand Power Snatch	40	1	6	perform for each arm
		50	1	6	
	Close Grip Power Snatch	50	1	6	
		60	1	6	
	Rx Squat	n/a	2	1	
	Pipeline Stretch	n/a	2	10	
	Drop Snatch	40	1	6	
		50	2	6	
		60	1	6	
	Bent Press w/Kbell	40	1	3	perform for each arm
		50	2	3	
		60	1	3	
	1 leg Good Morning	75	3	12	
	Towel Chins	75	3	12	

Section E	Activity	%E	#S	#R	Notes
	Leg Raise Pike		1	6	
	Leg Raise Tuck		1	6	
	Plank		2		30 Seconds
	Side Plank		2		30 Seconds
	Janda		2	3-5	

Commentary on Injuries/Muscle Fatigue/Diet

Week One • Day Two • Sections ABC

Section A	Activity	%E	#S	#R	Notes
Mobility Work	Tumbling		3		
	Dynamic hurdles:				3 set x 5 hurdles
	• Right knee over		3	5	
	• Left knee over		3	5	
	• Down center		3	5	
	Rope routine				
Sprints	Circuit A	65			Rest is 90 seconds
GPP	None				

Section B	Activity	%E	#S	#R	Notes
None					

Section C	Activity	%E	#S	#R	Notes
Med ball Circuit					Perform 2 Circuits

Key code: % E: percent of effort, # S: number of sets, # R: number of reps

Week One • Day Two • Sections DE

Section D	Activity	%E	#S	#R	Notes
None					

Section E	Activity	%E	#S	#R	Notes
None					

Commentary on Injuries/Muscle Fatigue/Diet

_____
_____
_____
_____
_____
_____
_____
_____
_____

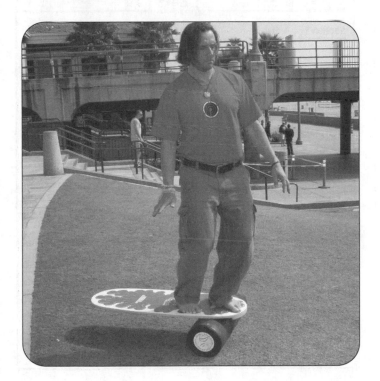

Week One • Day Three • Sections ABC

Section A	Activity	%E	#S	#R	Notes
Mobility Work	Tumbling		3		
	Dynamic hurdles:				3 set x 5 hurdles
	• Right knee over		3	5	
	• Left knee over		3	5	
	• Down center		3	5	
	Rope routine				
Sprints	None				
GPP	Sequence A		3		

Section B	Activity	%E	#S	#R	Notes
Quasi SPP	Balance Board				continuous motion
	Squats				30 seconds
	Ollie's		5	5	
	Shuv-its		5	5	
	Cut Back				30 seconds
	Surf - Only				
	Pop-Up		5		
	Hang 10's				30 seconds
	BoardWalks				30 seconds
	Pipeline				30 seconds
	Swiss Ball				
	Ball Dribbles				15 seconds
	Squats				30 seconds
	Back & Forth				30 seconds
	Outside Edge Roll				30 seconds

Repeat above sequence for 3 sets

Section C	Activity	%E	#S	#R	Notes
None					

Key code: % E: percent of effort, # S: number of sets, # R: number of reps

Week One • Day Three • Sections DE

Section D	Activity	%E	#S	#R	Notes
	Iron Cross	30	2	15	Rest is 60 seconds between sets
	Kettlebell Swings	30	2	15	
	Renegade Squat/Pull	30	2	15	
	Bench Press	40	1	6	
		50	2	6	
		60	1	6	
	Rx Squat	n/a	2	1	
	Pipeline Stretch	n/a	2	10	
	Squat/Push Press Com.	40	1	6	
		50	2	6	
		60	1	6	
	Shoulder Press	40	1	3	
		50	2	6	
		60	1	6	
	Natural Glute Ham	n/a	3	5	
	Bradford Press	75	3	12	

Section E	Activity	%E	#S	#R	Notes
	Leg Raise Pike		1	6	
	Leg Raise Tuck		1	6	
	Plank		2		30 Seconds
	Side Plank		2		30 Seconds
	Janda		2	3-5	

Commentary on Injuries/Muscle Fatigue/Diet

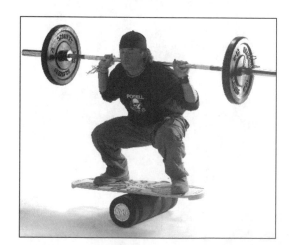

Week One • Day Four • Sections ABC

Section A	Activity	%E	#S	#R	Notes
Mobility Work	Tumbling		3		
	Dynamic hurdles:				3 set x 5 hurdles
	• Right knee over		3	5	
	• Left knee over		3	5	
	• Down center		3	5	
	Rope routine				
Sprints	Circuit B	65			Rest is 90 seconds
GPP	Sequence B		4		

Section B	Activity	%E	#S	#R	Notes
None					

Section C	Activity	%E	#S	#R	Notes
Med ball Circuit					Perform 2 Circuits

Key code: % E: percent of effort, # S: number of sets, # R: number of reps

Week One • Day Four • Sections DE

Section D	Activity	%E	#S	#R	Notes
None					

Section E	Activity	%E	#S	#R	Notes
None					

Commentary on Injuries/Muscle Fatigue/Diet

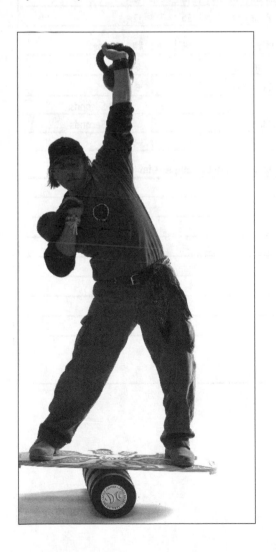

R

Week One • Day Five • Sections ABC

Section A	Activity	%E	#S	#R	Notes
Mobility Work	Tumbling		3		
	Dynamic hurdles:				3 set x 5 hurdles
	• Right knee over		3	5	
	• Left knee over		3	5	
	• Down center		3	5	
	Rope routine				
Sprints	Sequence B				
GPP	None				

Section B	Activity	%E	#S	#R	Notes
Quasi SPP	Balance Board				continuous motion
	Squats				30 seconds
	Ollie's		5	5	
	Shuv-its		5	5	
	Cut Back				30 seconds
	Surf - Only				
	Pop-Up		5		
	Hang 10's				30 seconds
	BoardWalks				30 seconds
	Pipeline				30 seconds
	Swiss Ball				
	Ball Dribbles				15 seconds
	Squats				30 seconds
	Back & Forth				30 seconds
	Outside Edge Roll				30 seconds
	Repeat above sequence for 3 sets				

Section C	Activity	%E	#S	#R	Notes
None					

Key code: % E: percent of effort, # S: number of sets, # R: number of reps

Week One • Day Five • Sections DE

Section D	Activity	%E	#S	#R	Notes
	Iron Cross	30	2	15	Rest is 60 seconds between sets
	Kettlebell Swings	30	2	15	
	Renegade Squat/Pull	30	2	15	
	1 Hand Power Clean	40	1	6	
		50	2	6	
		60	1	6	
	Rx Squat	n/a	2	1	
	Pipeline Stretch	n/a	2	10	
	Zercher Squat	40	1	6	
		50	2	6	
		60	1	6	
	Side Press w/Kbell	40	1	6	Perform for each arm
		50	2	6	
		60	2	6	
	Zercher Good Morning	75	3	12	
	Plate Raises	75	3	12	

Section E	Activity	%E	#S	#R	Notes
	Leg Raise Pike		1	6	
	Leg Raise Tuck		1	6	
	Plank		2		30 Seconds
	Side Plank		2		30 Seconds
	Janda		2	3-5	

Commentary on Injuries/Muscle Fatigue/Diet

_____

_____

_____

_____

_____

_____

_____

_____

_____

—Week Two—

Week Two • Day One • Sections ABC

Section A	Activity	%E	#S	#R	Notes
Mobility Work	Tumbling		3		
	Dynamic hurdles:				3 set x 5 hurdles
	• Right knee over		3	5	
	• Left knee over		3	5	
	• Down center		3	5	
	Rope routine				
Sprints	Sequence A		5		
GPP	Sequence A				

Section B	Activity	%E	#S	#R	Notes
Quasi SPP	Balance Board				continuous motion
	Squats				30 seconds
	Ollie's		5	5	
	Shuv-its		5	5	
	Cut Back				30 seconds
	Surf - Only				
	Pop-Up		5		
	Hang 10's				30 seconds
	BoardWalks				30 seconds
	Pipeline				30 seconds
	Swiss Ball				
	Ball Dribbles				15 seconds
	Squats				30 seconds
	Back & Forth				30 seconds
	Outside Edge Roll				30 seconds
	Repeat above sequence for 3 sets				

Section C	Activity	%E	#S	#R	Notes
None					

Key code: % E: percent of effort, # S: number of sets, # R: number of reps

Week Two • Day One • Sections DE

Section D	Activity	%E	#S	#R	Notes
	Iron Cross	30	2	15	**Rest is 60 seconds between sets**
	Kettlebell Swings	30	2	15	
	Renegade Squat/Pull	30	2	15	
	Cross-over Power Snatch	40	1	6	perform for each arm
		50	1	6	
	Close Grip Power Snatch	60	2	6	
	Rx Squat	n/a	2	1	
	Pipeline Stretch	n/a	2	10	
	Drop Snatch	40	1	6	
		50	1	6	
		60	2	6	
	Bent Press w/Kbell	40	1	3	perform for each arm
		50	1	3	
		60	2	3	
	1 leg Good Morning	75	3	12	
	Towel Chins	75	3	12	

Section E	Activity	%E	#S	#R	Notes
	Leg Raise Pike		1	6	
	Leg Raise Tuck		1	6	
	Plank		2		30 Seconds
	Side Plank		2		30 Seconds
	Janda		2	3-5	

Commentary on Injuries/Muscle Fatigue/Diet

Week Two • Day Two • Sections ABC

Section A	Activity	%E	#S	#R	Notes
Mobility Work	Tumbling		3		
	Dynamic hurdles:				3 set x 5 hurdles
	• Right knee over		3	5	
	• Left knee over		3	5	
	• Down center		3	5	
	Rope routine				
Sprints	Circuit A	65			Rest is 75 seconds
GPP	None		4		

Section B	Activity	%E	#S	#R	Notes
None					

Section C	Activity	%E	#S	#R	Notes
Med ball Circuit					Perform 2 Circuits

Key code: % E: percent of effort, # S: number of sets, # R: number of reps

Week Two • Day Two • Sections DE

Section D	Activity	%E	#S	#R	Notes
None					

Section E	Activity	%E	#S	#R	Notes
None					

Commentary on Injuries/Muscle Fatigue/Diet

_____

_____

_____

_____

_____

_____

_____

_____

_____

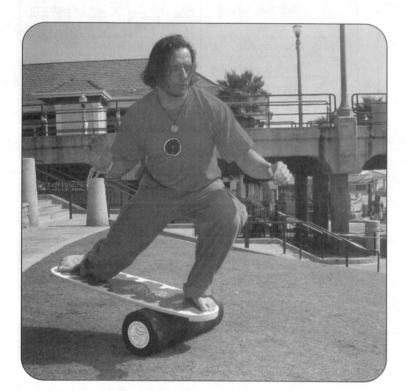

Week Two • Day Three • Sections ABC

Section A	Activity	%E	#S	#R	Notes
Mobility Work	Tumbling		3		
	Dynamic hurdles:				3 set x 5 hurdles
	• Right knee over		3	5	
	• Left knee over		3	5	
	• Down center		3	5	
	Rope routine				
Sprints	None				
GPP	Sequence A		4		

Section B	Activity	%E	#S	#R	Notes
Quasi SPP	Balance Board				continuous motion
	Squats				30 seconds
	Ollie's		5	5	
	Shuv-its		5	5	
	Cut Back				30 seconds
	Surf - Only				
	Pop-Up		5		
	Hang 10's				30 seconds
	BoardWalks				30 seconds
	Pipeline				30 seconds
	Swiss Ball				
	Ball Dribbles				15 seconds
	Squats				30 seconds
	Back & Forth				30 seconds
	Outside Edge Roll				30 seconds

Repeat above sequence for 3 sets

Section C	Activity	%E	#S	#R	Notes
None					

Key code: % E: percent of effort, # S: number of sets, # R: number of reps

Week Two • Day Three • Sections DE

Section D	Activity	%E	#S	#R	Notes
	Iron Cross	30	2	15	Rest is 60 seconds between sets
	Kettlebell Swings	30	2	15	
	Renegade Squat/Pull	30	2	15	
	Bench Press	40	1	6	perform for each arm
		50	1	6	
		60	2	6	
	Rx Squat	n/a	2	1	
	Pipeline Stretch	n/a	2	10	
	Squat	40	1	6	
		50	1	6	
		60	2	6	
	Push Press	40	1	6	perform for each arm
		50	1	6	
		60	2	6	
	Natural Glute Ham	n/a	3	5	
	Bradford Press	75	3	12	

Section E	Activity	%E	#S	#R	Notes
	Leg Raise Pike		1	6	
	Leg Raise Tuck		1	6	
	Plank		2		30 Seconds
	Side Plank		2		30 Seconds
	Janda		2	3-5	

Commentary on Injuries/Muscle Fatigue/Diet

Week Two • Day Four • Sections ABC

Section A	Activity	%E	#S	#R	Notes
Mobility Work	Tumbling		3		
	Dynamic hurdles:				3 set x 5 hurdles
	• Right knee over		3	5	
	• Left knee over		3	5	
	• Down center		3	5	
	Rope routine				
Sprints	Circuit B	65	3		Rest is 75 seconds
GPP	Sequence B				

Section B	Activity	%E	#S	#R	Notes
None					

Section C	Activity	%E	#S	#R	Notes
Med ball Circuit					Perform 2 Circuits

Key code: % E: percent of effort, # S: number of sets, # R: number of reps

Week Two • Day Four • Sections DE

Section D	Activity	%E	#S	#R	Notes
None					

Section E	Activity	%E	#S	#R	Notes
None					

Commentary on Injuries/Muscle Fatigue/Diet

_____
_____
_____
_____
_____
_____
_____
_____

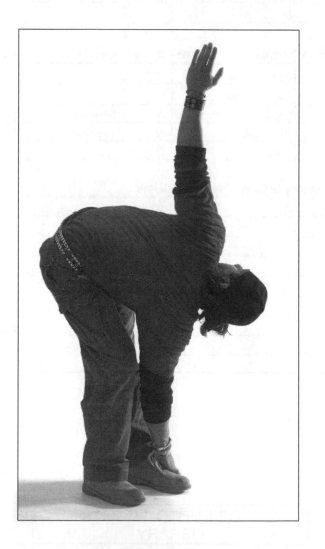

Week Two • Day Five • Sections ABC

Section A	Activity	%E	#S	#R	Notes
Mobility Work	Tumbling		3		
	Dynamic hurdles:				3 set x 5 hurdles
	• Right knee over		3	5	
	• Left knee over		3	5	
	• Down center		3	5	
	Rope routine				
Sprints	Sequence B				
GPP	None				

Section B	Activity	%E	#S	#R	Notes
Quasi SPP	Balance Board				continuous motion
	Squats				30 seconds
	Ollie's		5	5	
	Shuv-its		5	5	
	Cut Back				30 seconds
	Surf - Only				
	Pop-Up		5		
	Hang 10's				30 seconds
	BoardWalks				30 seconds
	Pipeline				30 seconds
	Swiss Ball				
	Ball Dribbles				15 seconds
	Squats				30 seconds
	Back & Forth				30 seconds
	Outside Edge Roll				30 seconds

Repeat above sequence for 3 sets

Section C	Activity	%E	#S	#R	Notes
None					

Key code: % E: percent of effort, # S: number of sets, # R: number of reps

Week Two • Day Five • Sections DE

Section D	Activity	%E	#S	#R	Notes
	Iron Cross	30	2	15	Rest is 60 seconds between sets
	Kettlebell Swings	30	2	15	
	Renegade Squat/Pull	30	2	15	
	Power Clean Hang or..	40	1	6	..."The Bear" complex
		50	1	6	...if Technique is good
		60	2	6	
	Rx Squat	n/a	2	1	
	Pipeline Stretch	n/a	2	10	
	Front Squat	40	1	6	
		50	1	6	
		60	2	6	
	See Saw w/ KBell	40	1	6	
		50	1	6	
		60	2	6	
	Zercher Good Morning	75	3	12	
	Plate Raises	75	3	12	

Section E	Activity	%E	#S	#R	Notes
	Leg Raise Pike		1	6	
	Leg Raise Tuck		1	6	
	Plank		2		30 Seconds
	Side Plank		2		30 Seconds
	Janda		2	3-5	

Commentary on Injuries/Muscle Fatigue/Diet

—Week Three—

Week Three • Day One • Sections ABC

Section A	Activity	%E	#S	#R	Notes
Mobility Work	Tumbling		3		
	Dynamic hurdles:				3 set x 5 hurdles
	• Right knee over		3	5	
	• Left knee over		3	5	
	• Down center		3	5	
	Rope routine				
Sprints	Sequence A				
GPP	Sequence A		4		

Section B	Activity	%E	#S	#R	Notes
Quasi SPP	Balance Board				continuous motion
	Squats				30 seconds
	Ollie's		5	5	
	Shuv-its		5	5	
	Cut Back				30 seconds
	Surf - Only				
	Pop-Up		5		
	Hang 10's				30 seconds
	BoardWalks				30 seconds
	Pipeline				30 seconds
	Swiss Ball				
	Ball Dribbles				15 seconds
	Squats				30 seconds
	Back & Forth				30 seconds
	Outside Edge Roll				30 seconds
	Repeat above sequence for 3 sets				

Section C	Activity	%E	#S	#R	Notes
None					

Key code: % E: percent of effort, # S: number of sets, # R: number of reps

Week Three • Day One • Sections DEF

Section D	Activity	%E	#S	#R	Notes
	Triple Jumps		2		
	Box Jump Up & Out		2		
	Barrier Jumps		2		

Section E	Activity	%E	#S	#R	Notes
	Iron Cross	30	2	15	**Rest is 60 seconds between sets**
	Kettlebell Swings	30	2	15	
	Renegade Squat/Pull	30	2	15	
	1 Hand Power Snatch	40	1	6	
		50	1	6	
		60	1	6	
	Rx Squat	n/a	2	1	
	Pipeline Stretch	n/a	2	10	
	Drop Snatch	40	1	6	
		50	1	6	
		60	2	6	
	Bent Press	40	1	3	Perform with each arm
		50	1	3	
		60	2	3	
	1 Leg Good Morning	75	3	12	
	Towel Chins	75	3	12	

Section F	Activity	%E	#S	#R	Notes
	Leg Raise Pike		1	6	
	Leg Raise Tuck		1	6	
	Plank		2		30 Seconds
	Side Plank		2		30 Seconds
	Janda		2	3-5	

Commentary on Injuries/Muscle Fatigue/Diet

_____

_____

_____

_____

R

Week Three • Day Two • Sections ABC

Section A	Activity	%E	#S	#R	Notes
Mobility Work	Tumbling		3		
	Dynamic hurdles:				3 set x 5 hurdles
	• Right knee over		3	5	
	• Left knee over		3	5	
	• Down center		3	5	
	Rope routine				
Sprints	Circuit A	65			Rest is 90 seconds
GPP	None				

Section B	Activity	%E	#S	#R	Notes
None					

Section C	Activity	%E	#S	#R	Notes
Med ball Circuit					Perform 2 Circuits

Key code: % E: percent of effort, # S: number of sets, # R: number of reps

Week Three • Day Two • Sections DEF

Section D	Activity	%E	#S	#R	Notes
None					

Section E	Activity	%E	#S	#R	Notes
None					

Section F	Activity	%E	#S	#R	Notes
None					

Commentary on Injuries/Muscle Fatigue/Diet

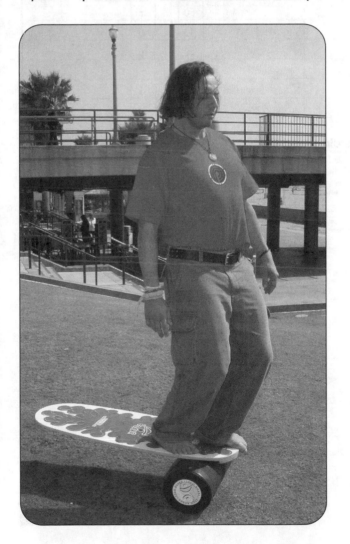

Week Three • Day Three • Sections ABC

Section A	Activity	%E	#S	#R	Notes
Mobility Work	Tumbling		3		
	Dynamic hurdles:				3 set x 5 hurdles
	• Right knee over		3	5	
	• Left knee over		3	5	
	• Down center		3	5	
	Rope routine				
Sprints	None				
GPP	Sequence A		3		

Section B	Activity	%E	#S	#R	Notes
Quasi SPP	Balance Board				continuous motion
	Squats				30 seconds
	Ollie's		5	5	
	Shuv-its		5	5	
	Cut Back				30 seconds
	Surf - Only				
	Pop-Up		5		
	Hang 10's				30 seconds
	BoardWalks				30 seconds
	Pipeline				30 seconds
	Swiss Ball				
	Ball Dribbles				15 seconds
	Squats				30 seconds
	Back & Forth				30 seconds
	Outside Edge Roll				30 seconds
	Repeat above sequence for 3 sets				

Section C	Activity	%E	#S	#R	Notes
None					

Key code: % E: percent of effort, # S: number of sets, # R: number of reps

Week Three • Day Three • Sections DEF

Section D	Activity	%E	#S	#R	Notes
	Triple Jumps		4		
	Box Jump Up & Out		4		
	Barrier Jumps		2		

Section E	Activity	%E	#S	#R	Notes
	Iron Cross	30	2	15	**Rest is 60 seconds between sets**
	Kettlebell Swings	30	2	15	
	Renegade Squat/Pull	30	2	15	
	Bench Press	40	1	6	
		50	1	6	
		60	1	6	
	Rx Squat	n/a	2	1	
	Pipeline Stretch	n/a	2	10	
	Squat/Push Press...	40	1	6	...Complex
		50	1	6	
		60	1	6	
	Shoulder Press	40	1	6	
		50	1	6	
		60	2	6	
	Natural Glute Ham	n/a	3	5	
	Bradford Press	75	3	12	

Section F	Activity	%E	#S	#R	Notes
	Leg Raise Pike		1	6	
	Leg Raise Tuck		1	6	
	Plank		2		30 Seconds
	Side Plank		2		30 Seconds
	Janda		2	3-5	

Commentary on Injuries/Muscle Fatigue/Diet

_____

_____

_____

_____

_____

_____

_____

_____

Week Three • Day Four • Sections ABC

Section A	Activity	%E	#S	#R	Notes
Mobility Work	Tumbling		3		
	Dynamic hurdles:				3 set x 5 hurdles
	• Right knee over		3	5	
	• Left knee over		3	5	
	• Down center		3	5	
	Rope routine				
Sprints	Circuit B	65			Rest is 75 seconds
GPP	Sequence B		4		

Section B	Activity	%E	#S	#R	Notes
None					

Section C	Activity	%E	#S	#R	Notes
Med ball Circuit					Perform 2 Circuits

Key code: % E: percent of effort, # S: number of sets, # R: number of reps

Week Three • Day Four • Sections DEF

Section D	Activity	%E	#S	#R	Notes
None					

Section E	Activity	%E	#S	#R	Notes
None					

Section F	Activity	%E	#S	#R	Notes
None					

Commentary on Injuries/Muscle Fatigue/Diet

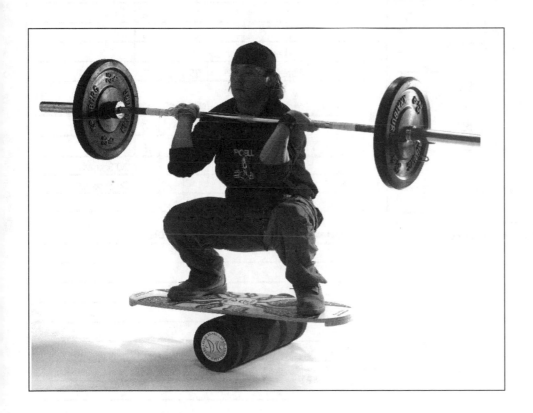

Week Three • Day Five • Sections ABC

Section A	Activity	%E	#S	#R	Notes
Mobility Work	Tumbling		3		
	Dynamic hurdles:				3 set x 5 hurdles
	• Right knee over		3	5	
	• Left knee over		3	5	
	• Down center		3	5	
	Rope routine				
Sprints	Sequence B				
GPP	None				

Section B	Activity	%E	#S	#R	Notes
Quasi SPP	Balance Board				continuous motion
	Squats				30 seconds
	Ollie's		5	5	
	Shuv-its		5	5	
	Cut Back				30 seconds
	Surf - Only				
	Pop-Up		5		
	Hang 10's				30 seconds
	BoardWalks				30 seconds
	Pipeline				30 seconds
	Swiss Ball				
	Ball Dribbles				15 seconds
	Squats				30 seconds
	Back & Forth				30 seconds
	Outside Edge Roll				30 seconds
	Repeat above sequence for 3 sets				

Section C	Activity	%E	#S	#R	Notes
None					

Key code: % E: percent of effort, # S: number of sets, # R: number of reps

Week Three • Day Five • Sections DEF

Section D	Activity	%E	#S	#R	Notes
	Triple Jumps		3		
	Box Jump Up & Out		3		
	Barrier Jumps		1		

Section E	Activity	%E	#S	#R	Notes
	Iron Cross	30	2	15	**Rest is 60 seconds between sets**
	Kettlebell Swings	30	2	15	
	Renegade Squat/Pull	30	2	15	
	1 Hand Power Clean or...	40	1	6	...'The Bear" complex
		50	1	6	...if Technique is good
		60	2	6	
	Rx Squat	n/a	2		
	Pipeline Stretch	n/a	2	10	
	Zercher Squat	40	1	6	
		50	1	6	
		60	1	6	
	Side Press	40	1	6	perform for each arm
		50	1	6	
		60	1	6	
	Zercher Good Morning	75	3	12	
	Plate Raises	75	3	12	

Section F	Activity	%E	#S	#R	Notes
	Leg Raise Pike		1	6	
	Leg Raise Tuck		1	6	
	Plank		2		30 Seconds
	Side Plank		2		30 Seconds
	Janda		2	3-5	

Commentary on Injuries/Muscle Fatigue/Diet

_____

_____

_____

_____

_____

_____

_____

_____

—Week Four—

Week Four • Day One • Sections ABC

Section A	Activity	%E	#S	#R	Notes
Mobility Work	Tumbling		3		
	Dynamic hurdles:				3 set x 5 hurdles
	• Right knee over		3	5	
	• Left knee over		3	5	
	• Down center		3	5	
	Rope routine				
Sprints	Sequence A				
GPP	Sequence A		5		

Section B	Activity	%E	#S	#R	Notes
Quasi SPP	Balance Board				continuous motion
	Squats				30 seconds
	Ollie's		5	5	
	Shuv-its		5	5	
	Cut Back				30 seconds
	Surf - Only				
	Pop-Up		5		
	Hang 10's				30 seconds
	BoardWalks				30 seconds
	Pipeline				30 seconds
	Swiss Ball				
	Ball Dribbles				15 seconds
	Squats				30 seconds
	Back & Forth				30 seconds
	Outside Edge Roll				30 seconds
	Repeat above sequence for 3 sets				

Section C	Activity	%E	#S	#R	Notes
None					

Key code: % E: percent of effort, # S: number of sets, # R: number of reps

Week Four • Day One • Sections DEF

Section D	Activity	%E	#S	#R	Notes
	Triple Jumps		3		
	Box Jump Up & Out		3		
	Barrier Jumps		2		

Section E	Activity	%E	#S	#R	Notes
	Iron Cross	30	2	15	**Rest is 60 seconds between sets**
	Kettlebell Swings	30	2	15	
	Renegade Squat/Pull	30	2	15	
	Crossover Power Snatch	45	1	6	
		55	1	6	
	Close Grip Power Snatch	65	2	6	
	Rx Squat	n/a	2	1	
	Pipeline Stretch	n/a	2	10	
	Drop Snatch	45	1	6	
		55	1	6	
		65	2	6	
	Bent Press	45	1	3	Perform with each arm
		55	1	3	
		65	2	3	
	1 Leg Good Morning	75	3	12	
	Towel Chins	75	3	12	

Section F	Activity	%E	#S	#R	Notes
	Leg Raise Pike		1	6	
	Leg Raise Tuck		1	6	
	Plank		2		30 Seconds
	Side Plank		2		30 Seconds
	Janda		2	3-5	

Commentary on Injuries/Muscle Fatigue/Diet

Week Four • Day Two • Sections ABC

Section A	Activity	%E	#S	#R	Notes
Mobility Work	Tumbling		3		
	Dynamic hurdles:				3 set x 5 hurdles
	• Right knee over		3	5	
	• Left knee over		3	5	
	• Down center		3	5	
	Rope routine				
Sprints	Circuit A	65			Rest is 60 seconds
GPP	None				

Section B	Activity	%E	#S	#R	Notes
None					

Section C	Activity	%E	#S	#R	Notes
Med ball Circuit					Perform 2 Circuits

Key code: % E: percent of effort, # S: number of sets, # R: number of reps

Week Four • Day Two • Sections DEF

Section D	Activity	%E	#S	#R	Notes
None					

Section E	Activity	%E	#S	#R	Notes
None					

Section F	Activity	%E	#S	#R	Notes
None					

Commentary on Injuries/Muscle Fatigue/Diet

_____

_____

_____

_____

_____

_____

_____

_____

_____

_____

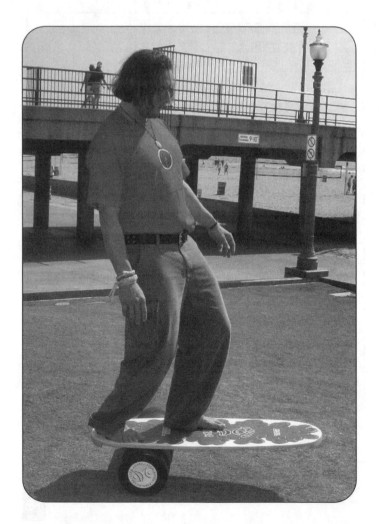

Week Four • Day Three • Sections ABC

Section A	Activity	%E	#S	#R	Notes
Mobility Work	Tumbling		3		
	Dynamic hurdles:				3 set x 5 hurdles
	• Right knee over		3	5	
	• Left knee over		3	5	
	• Down center		3	5	
	Rope routine				
Sprints	None				
GPP	Sequence A		3		

Section B	Activity	%E	#S	#R	Notes
Quasi SPP	Balance Board				continuous motion
	Squats				30 seconds
	Ollie's		5	5	
	Shuv-its		5	5	
	Cut Back				30 seconds
	Surf - Only				
	Pop-Up		5		
	Hang 10's				30 seconds
	BoardWalks				30 seconds
	Pipeline				30 seconds
	Swiss Ball				
	Ball Dribbles				15 seconds
	Squats				30 seconds
	Back & Forth				30 seconds
	Outside Edge Roll				30 seconds
	Repeat above sequence for 3 sets				

Section C	Activity	%E	#S	#R	Notes
None					

Key code: % E: percent of effort, # S: number of sets, # R: number of reps

Week Four • Day Three • Sections DEF

Section D	Activity	%E	#S	#R	Notes
	Triple Jumps		5		
	Box Jump Up & Out		5		
	Barrier Jumps		3		

Section E	Activity	%E	#S	#R	Notes
	Iron Cross	30	2	15	**Rest is 60 seconds between sets**
	Kettlebell Swings	30	2	15	
	Renegade Squat/Pull	30	2	15	
	Bench Press	45	1	6	
		55	1	6	
		65	2	6	
	Rx Squat	n/a	2	1	
	Pipeline Stretch	n/a	2	10	
	Squat	45	1	6	
		55	1	6	
		65	2	6	
	Push Press	45	1	6	
		55	1	6	
		65	2	6	
	Natural Glute Ham	n/a	3	5	
	Bradford Press	75	3	12	

Section F	Activity	%E	#S	#R	Notes
	Leg Raise Pike		1	6	
	Leg Raise Tuck		1	6	
	Plank		2		30 Seconds
	Side Plank		2		30 Seconds
	Janda		2	3-5	

Commentary on Injuries/Muscle Fatigue/Diet

Week Four • Day Four • Sections ABC

Section A	Activity	%E	#S	#R	Notes
Mobility Work	Tumbling		3		
	Dynamic hurdles:				3 set x 5 hurdles
	• Right knee over		3	5	
	• Left knee over		3	5	
	• Down center		3	5	
	Rope routine				
Sprints	Circuit B	65			Rest is 60 seconds
GPP	Sequence B		4		

Section B	Activity	%E	#S	#R	Notes
None					

Section C	Activity	%E	#S	#R	Notes
Med ball Circuit					Perform 2 Circuits

Key code: % E: percent of effort, # S: number of sets, # R: number of reps

Week Four • Day Four • Sections DEF

Section D	Activity	%E	#S	#R	Notes
None					

Section E	Activity	%E	#S	#R	Notes
None					

Section F	Activity	%E	#S	#R	Notes
None					

Commentary on Injuries/Muscle Fatigue/Diet

_____
_____
_____
_____
_____
_____
_____
_____
_____
_____

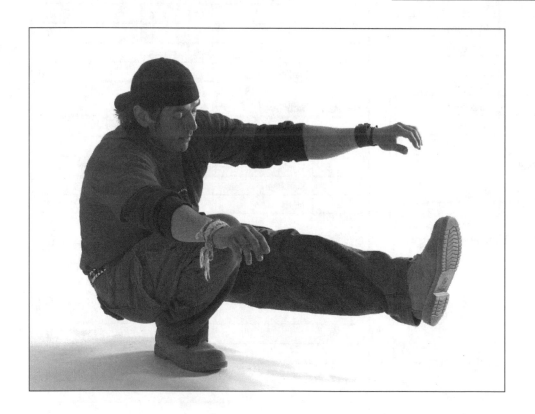

Week Four • Day Five • Sections ABC

Section A	Activity	%E	#S	#R	Notes
Mobility Work	Tumbling		3		
	Dynamic hurdles:				3 set x 5 hurdles
	• Right knee over		3	5	
	• Left knee over		3	5	
	• Down center		3	5	
	Rope routine				
Sprints	Sequence B				
GPP	None				

Section B	Activity	%E	#S	#R	Notes
Quasi SPP	Balance Board				continuous motion
	Squats				30 seconds
	Ollie's		5	5	
	Shuv-its		5	5	
	Cut Back				30 seconds
	Surf - Only				
	Pop-Up		5		
	Hang 10's				30 seconds
	BoardWalks				30 seconds
	Pipeline				30 seconds
	Swiss Ball				
	Ball Dribbles				15 seconds
	Squats				30 seconds
	Back & Forth				30 seconds
	Outside Edge Roll				30 seconds
	Repeat above sequence for 3 sets				

Section C	Activity	%E	#S	#R	Notes
None					

Key code: % E: percent of effort, # S: number of sets, # R: number of reps

Week Four • Day Five • Sections DEF

Section D	Activity	%E	#S	#R	Notes
	Triple Jumps		2		
	Box Jump Up & Out		2		
	Barrier Jumps		2		

Section E	Activity	%E	#S	#R	Notes
	Iron Cross	30	2	15	**Rest is 60 seconds between sets**
	Kettlebell Swings	30	2	15	
	Renegade Squat/Pull	30	2	15	
	Power Clean Hang or..	45	1	6	..."The Bear" complex
		55	1	6	...if Technique is good
		65	2	6	
	Rx Squat	n/a	2	1	
	Pipeline Stretch	n/a	2	10	
	Front Squat	45	1	6	
		55	1	6	
		65	1	6	
	SeeSaw w/ Kbell	45	1	6	perform for each arm
		55	1	6	
		65	1	6	
	Zercher Good Morning	75	3	12	
	Plate Raises	75	3	12	

Section F	Activity	%E	#S	#R	Notes
	Leg Raise Pike		1	6	
	Leg Raise Tuck		1	6	
	Plank		2		30 Seconds
	Side Plank		2		30 Seconds
	Janda		2	3-5	

Commentary on Injuries/Muscle Fatigue/Diet

_____

_____

_____

_____

_____

_____

_____

_____

_____

—Week Five—

Week Five • Day One • Sections ABC

Section A	Activity	%E	#S	#R	Notes
Mobility Work	Tumbling		3		
	Dynamic hurdles:				3 set x 5 hurdles
	• Right knee over		3	5	
	• Left knee over		3	5	
	• Down center		3	5	
	Rope routine				
Sprints	Sequence A				
GPP	None				

Section B	Activity	%E	#S	#R	Notes
Quasi SPP	Balance Board				continuous motion
	Squats				30 seconds
	Ollie's		5	5	
	Shuv-its		5	5	
	Cut Back				30 seconds
	Surf - Only				
	Pop-Up		5		
	Hang 10's				30 seconds
	BoardWalks				30 seconds
	Pipeline				30 seconds
	Swiss Ball				
	Ball Dribbles				15 seconds
	Squats				30 seconds
	Back & Forth				30 seconds
	Outside Edge Roll				30 seconds
	Repeat above sequence for 3 sets				

Section C	Activity	%E	#S	#R	Notes
None					

Key code: % E: percent of effort, # S: number of sets, # R: number of reps

Week Five • Day One • Sections DEF

Section D	Activity	%E	#S	#R	Notes
	Triple Jumps		2		
	Box Jump Up & Out		2		
	Barrier Jumps		2		

Section E	Activity	%E	#S	#R	Notes
	Iron Cross	30	2	15	Rest is 60 seconds between sets
	Kettlebell Swings	30	2	15	
	Renegade Squat/Pull	30	2	15	
	Squat/Burpee Complex	50	1	6	
		60	1	6	
		65	2	6	
	Rx Squat	n/a	2	1	
	Pipeline Stretch	n/a	2	10	
	Drop Snatch	50	1	6	
		60	1	6	
		65	2	6	
	Bent Press	50	1	3	Perform with each arm
		60	1	3	
		65	2	3	
	1 Leg Good Morning	75	3	12	
	Towel Chins	75	3	12	

Section F	Activity	%E	#S	#R	Notes
	Leg Raise Pike		1	6	
	Leg Raise Tuck		1	6	
	Plank		2		30 Seconds
	Side Plank		2		30 Seconds
	Janda		2	3-5	

Commentary on Injuries/Muscle Fatigue/Diet

_____

_____

_____

_____

_____

Week Five • Day Two • Sections ABC

Section A	Activity	%E	#S	#R	Notes
Mobility Work	Tumbling		3		
	Dynamic hurdles:				3 set x 5 hurdles
	• Right knee over		3	5	
	• Left knee over		3	5	
	• Down center		3	5	
	Rope routine				
Sprints	Circuit A	65			Rest is 45 seconds
GPP	None				

Section B	Activity	%E	#S	#R	Notes
None					

Section C	Activity	%E	#S	#R	Notes
Med ball Circuit					Perform 2 Circuits

Key code: % E: percent of effort, # S: number of sets, # R: number of reps

Week Five • Day Two • Sections DEF

Section D	Activity	%E	#S	#R	Notes
None					

Section E	Activity	%E	#S	#R	Notes
None					

Section F	Activity	%E	#S	#R	Notes
None					

Commentary on Injuries/Muscle Fatigue/Diet

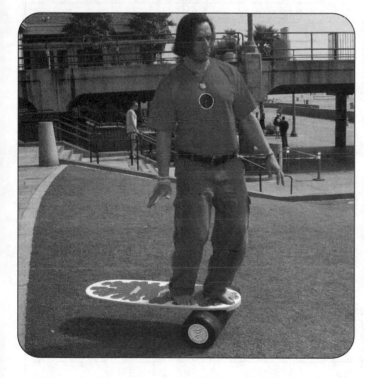

Week Five • Day Three • Sections ABC

Section A	Activity	%E	#S	#R	Notes
Mobility Work	Tumbling		3		
	Dynamic hurdles:				3 set x 5 hurdles
	• Right knee over		3	5	
	• Left knee over		3	5	
	• Down center		3	5	
	Rope routine				
Sprints	None				
GPP	None				

Section B	Activity	%E	#S	#R	Notes
Quasi SPP	Balance Board				continuous motion
	Squats				30 seconds
	Ollie's		5	5	
	Shuv-its		5	5	
	Cut Back				30 seconds
	Surf - Only				
	Pop-Up		5		
	Hang 10's				30 seconds
	BoardWalks				30 seconds
	Pipeline				30 seconds
	Swiss Ball				
	Ball Dribbles				15 seconds
	Squats				30 seconds
	Back & Forth				30 seconds
	Outside Edge Roll				30 seconds

Repeat above sequence for 3 sets

Section C	Activity	%E	#S	#R	Notes
None					

Key code: % E: percent of effort, # S: number of sets, # R: number of reps

Week Five • Day Three • Sections DEF

Section D	Activity	%E	#S	#R	Notes
	Triple Jumps		4		
	Box Jump Up & Out		4		
	Barrier Jumps		3		

Section E	Activity	%E	#S	#R	Notes
	Iron Cross	30	2	15	**Rest is 60 seconds between sets**
	Kettlebell Swings	30	2	15	
	Renegade Squat/Pull	30	2	15	
	Bench Press	50	1	6	
		60	1	6	
		65	2	6	
	Rx Squat	n/a	2	1	
	Pipeline Stretch	n/a	2	10	
	Squat/Push Press...	50	1	6	...Complex
		60	1	6	
		65	2	6	
	Shoulder Press	45	1	6	
		55	1	6	
		65	2	6	
	Natural Glute Ham	n/a	3	5	
	Bradford Press	75	3	12	

Section F	Activity	%E	#S	#R	Notes
	Leg Raise Pike		1	6	
	Leg Raise Tuck		1	6	
	Plank		2		30 Seconds
	Side Plank		2		30 Seconds
	Janda		2	3-5	

Commentary on Injuries/Muscle Fatigue/Diet

Week Five • Day Four • Sections ABC

Section A	Activity	%E	#S	#R	Notes
Mobility Work	Tumbling		3		
	Dynamic hurdles:				3 set x 5 hurdles
	• Right knee over		3	5	
	• Left knee over		3	5	
	• Down center		3	5	
	Rope routine				
Sprints	Circuit B	65			Rest is 45 seconds
GPP	None				

Section B	Activity	%E	#S	#R	Notes
None					

Section C	Activity	%E	#S	#R	Notes
Med ball Circuit					Perform 2 Circuits

Key code: % E: percent of effort, # S: number of sets, # R: number of reps

Week Five • Day Four • Sections DEF

Section D	Activity	%E	#S	#R	Notes
None					

Section E	Activity	%E	#S	#R	Notes
None					

Section F	Activity	%E	#S	#R	Notes
None					

Commentary on Injuries/Muscle Fatigue/Diet

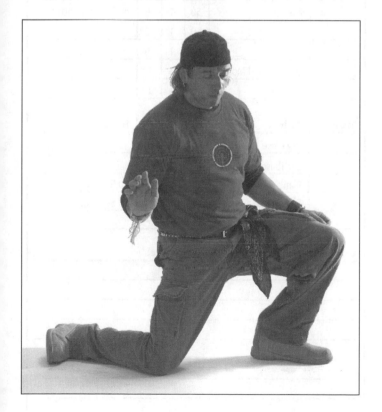

Week Five • Day Five • Sections ABC

Section A	Activity	%E	#S	#R	Notes
Mobility Work	Tumbling		3		
	Dynamic hurdles:				3 set x 5 hurdles
	• Right knee over		3	5	
	• Left knee over		3	5	
	• Down center		3	5	
	Rope routine				
Sprints	Sequence B				
GPP	None				

Section B	Activity	%E	#S	#R	Notes
Quasi SPP	Balance Board				continuous motion
	Squats				30 seconds
	Ollie's		5	5	
	Shuv-its		5	5	
	Cut Back				30 seconds
	Surf - Only				
	Pop-Up		5		
	Hang 10's				30 seconds
	BoardWalks				30 seconds
	Pipeline				30 seconds
	Swiss Ball				
	Ball Dribbles				15 seconds
	Squats				30 seconds
	Back & Forth				30 seconds
	Outside Edge Roll				30 seconds
	Repeat above sequence for 3 sets				

Section C	Activity	%E	#S	#R	Notes
None					

Key code: % E: percent of effort, # S: number of sets, # R: number of reps

Week Five • Day Five • Sections DEF

Section D	Activity	%E	#S	#R	Notes
	Triple Jumps		3		
	Box Jump Up & Out		3		
	Barrier Jumps		1		

Section E	Activity	%E	#S	#R	Notes
	Iron Cross	30	2	15	**Rest is 60 seconds between sets**
	Kettlebell Swings	30	2	15	
	Renegade Squat/Pull	30	2	15	
	The Bear	50	1	6	
		60	1	6	
		65	2	6	
	Rx Squat	n/a	2	1	
	Pipeline Stretch	n/a	2	10	
	Zercher Squat	50	1	6	
		60	1	6	
		65	2	6	
	Side Press	50	1	6	perform for each arm
		60	1	6	
		65	1	6	
	Zercher Good Morning	75	3	12	
	Plate Raises	75	3	12	

Section F	Activity	%E	#S	#R	Notes
	Leg Raise Pike		1	6	
	Leg Raise Tuck		1	6	
	Plank		2		30 Seconds
	Side Plank		2		30 Seconds
	Janda		2	3-5	

Commentary on Injuries/Muscle Fatigue/Diet

_____

_____

_____

_____

_____

_____

_____

_____

—Week Six—

Week Six • Day One • Sections ABC

Section A	Activity	%E	#S	#R	Notes
Mobility Work	Tumbling		3		
	Dynamic hurdles:				3 set x 5 hurdles
	• Right knee over		3	5	
	• Left knee over		3	5	
	• Down center		3	5	
	Rope routine				
Sprints	Sequence A				
GPP	None				

Section B	Activity	%E	#S	#R	Notes
Quasi SPP	Balance Board				continuous motion
	Squats				30 seconds
	Ollie's		5	5	
	Shuv-its		5	5	
	Cut Back				30 seconds
	Surf - Only				
	Pop-Up		5		
	Hang 10's				30 seconds
	BoardWalks				30 seconds
	Pipeline				30 seconds
	Swiss Ball				
	Ball Dribbles				15 seconds
	Squats				30 seconds
	Back & Forth				30 seconds
	Outside Edge Roll				30 seconds

Repeat above sequence for 3 sets

Section C	Activity	%E	#S	#R	Notes
None					

Key code: % E: percent of effort, # S: number of sets, # R: number of reps

Week Six • Day One • Sections DEF

Section D	Activity	%E	#S	#R	Notes
	Triple Jumps		2		
	Box Jump Up & Out		2		
	Barrier Jumps		2		

Section E	Activity	%E	#S	#R	Notes
	Iron Cross	30	2	15	**Rest is 60 seconds between sets**
	Kettlebell Swings	30	2	15	
	Renegade Squat/Pull	30	2	15	
	Squat/Burpee Complex	60	2	6	
		65	2	6	
	Rx Squat	n/a	2	1	
	Pipeline Stretch	n/a	2	10	
	Drop Snatch	60	2	6	
		65	2	6	
	Bent Press	60	2	3	Perform with each arm
		65	2	3	
	1 Leg Good Morning	75	3	12	
	Towel Chins	75	3	12	

Section F	Activity	%E	#S	#R	Notes
	Leg Raise Pike		1	6	
	Leg Raise Tuck		1	6	
	Plank		2		30 Seconds
	Side Plank		2		30 Seconds
	Janda		2	3-5	

Commentary on Injuries/Muscle Fatigue/Diet

_____

_____

_____

_____

_____

_____

_____

Week Six • Day Two • Sections ABC

Section A	Activity	%E	#S	#R	Notes
Mobility Work	Tumbling		3		
	Dynamic hurdles:				3 set x 5 hurdles
	• Right knee over		3	5	
	• Left knee over		3	5	
	• Down center		3	5	
	Rope routine				
Sprints	Circuit A	65			Rest is 60 seconds
GPP	None				

Section B	Activity	%E	#S	#R	Notes
None					

Section C	Activity	%E	#S	#R	Notes
Med ball Circuit					Perform 2 Circuits

Key code: % E: percent of effort, # S: number of sets, # R: number of reps

Week Six • Day Two • Sections DEF

Section D	Activity	%E	#S	#R	Notes
None					

Section E	Activity	%E	#S	#R	Notes
None					

Section F	Activity	%E	#S	#R	Notes
None					

Commentary on Injuries/Muscle Fatigue/Diet

_____
_____
_____
_____
_____
_____
_____
_____
_____
_____

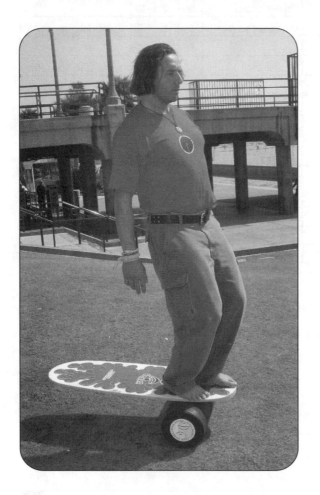

Week Six • Day Three • Sections ABC

Section A	Activity	%E	#S	#R	Notes
Mobility Work	Tumbling		3		
	Dynamic hurdles:				3 set x 5 hurdles
	• Right knee over		3	5	
	• Left knee over		3	5	
	• Down center		3	5	
	Rope routine				
Sprints	None				
GPP	None				

Section B	Activity	%E	#S	#R	Notes
Quasi SPP	Balance Board				continuous motion
	Squats				30 seconds
	Ollie's		5	5	
	Shuv-its		5	5	
	Cut Back				30 seconds
	Surf - Only				
	Pop-Up		5		
	Hang 10's				30 seconds
	BoardWalks				30 seconds
	Pipeline				30 seconds
	Swiss Ball				
	Ball Dribbles				15 seconds
	Squats				30 seconds
	Back & Forth				30 seconds
	Outside Edge Roll				30 seconds

Repeat above sequence for 3 sets

Section C	Activity	%E	#S	#R	Notes
None					

Key code: % E: percent of effort, # S: number of sets, # R: number of reps

Week Six • Day Three • Sections DEF

Section D	Activity	%E	#S	#R	Notes
	Triple Jumps		4		
	Box Jump Up & Out		4		
	Barrier Jumps		3		

Section E	Activity	%E	#S	#R	Notes
	Iron Cross	30	2	15	**Rest is 60 seconds between sets**
	Kettlebell Swings	30	2	15	
	Renegade Squat/Pull	30	2	15	
	Bench Press	60	2	6	
		65	2	6	
	Rx Squat	n/a	2	1	
	Pipeline Stretch	n/a	2	10	
	Squat/Push Press...	60	2	6	...Complex
		65	2	6	
	Shoulder Press	60	2	6	
		65	2	6	
	Natural Glute Ham	75	3	5	
	Bradford Press	75	3	12	

Section F	Activity	%E	#S	#R	Notes
	Leg Raise Pike		1	6	
	Leg Raise Tuck		1	6	
	Plank		2		30 Seconds
	Side Plank		2		30 Seconds
	Janda		2	3-5	

Commentary on Injuries/Muscle Fatigue/Diet

_____

_____

_____

_____

_____

_____

_____

_____

_____

Week Six • Day Four • Sections ABC

Section A	Activity	%E	#S	#R	Notes
Mobility Work	Tumbling		3		
	Dynamic hurdles:				3 set x 5 hurdles
	• Right knee over		3	5	
	• Left knee over		3	5	
	• Down center		3	5	
	Rope routine				
Sprints	Circuit B	65			Rest is 60 seconds
GPP	None				

Section B	Activity	%E	#S	#R	Notes
None					

Section C	Activity	%E	#S	#R	Notes
Med ball Circuit					Perform 2 Circuits

Key code: % E: percent of effort, # S: number of sets, # R: number of reps

Week Six • Day Four • Sections DEF

Section D	Activity	%E	#S	#R	Notes
None					

Section E	Activity	%E	#S	#R	Notes
None					

Section F	Activity	%E	#S	#R	Notes
None					

Commentary on Injuries/Muscle Fatigue/Diet

_____

_____

_____

_____

_____

_____

_____

_____

_____

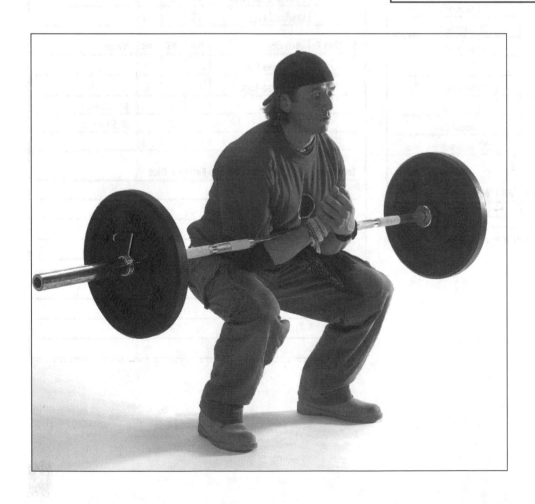

Week Six • Day Five • Sections ABC

Section A	Activity	%E	#S	#R	Notes
Mobility Work	Tumbling		3		
	Dynamic hurdles:				3 set x 5 hurdles
	• Right knee over		3	5	
	• Left knee over		3	5	
	• Down center		3	5	
	Rope routine				
Sprints	Sequence B				
GPP	None				

Section B	Activity	%E	#S	#R	Notes
Quasi SPP	Balance Board				continuous motion
	Squats				30 seconds
	Ollie's		5	5	
	Shuv-its		5	5	
	Cut Back				30 seconds
	Surf - Only				
	Pop-Up		5		
	Hang 10's				30 seconds
	BoardWalks				30 seconds
	Pipeline				30 seconds
	Swiss Ball				
	Ball Dribbles				15 seconds
	Squats				30 seconds
	Back & Forth				30 seconds
	Outside Edge Roll				30 seconds
	Repeat above sequence for 3 sets				

Section C	Activity	%E	#S	#R	Notes
None					

Key code: % E: percent of effort, # S: number of sets, # R: number of reps

Week Six • Day Five • Sections DEF

Section D	Activity	%E	#S	#R	Notes
	Triple Jumps		3		
	Box Jump Up & Out		3		
	Barrier Jumps		1		

Section E	Activity	%E	#S	#R	Notes
	Iron Cross	30	2	15	**Rest is 60 seconds between sets**
	Kettlebell Swings	30	2	15	
	Renegade Squat/Pull	30	2	15	
	The Bear	60	2	6	
		65	2	6	
	Rx Squat	n/a	2	1	
	Pipeline Stretch	n/a	2	10	
	Zercher Squat	60	2	6	
		65	2	6	
	Side Press	60	2	6	perform for each arm
		65	2	6	
	Zercher Good Morning	75	3	12	
	Plate Raises	75	3	12	

Section F	Activity	%E	#S	#R	Notes
	Leg Raise Pike		1	6	
	Leg Raise Tuck		1	6	
	Plank		2		30 Seconds
	Side Plank		2		30 Seconds
	Janda		2	3-5	

Commentary on Injuries/Muscle Fatigue/Diet

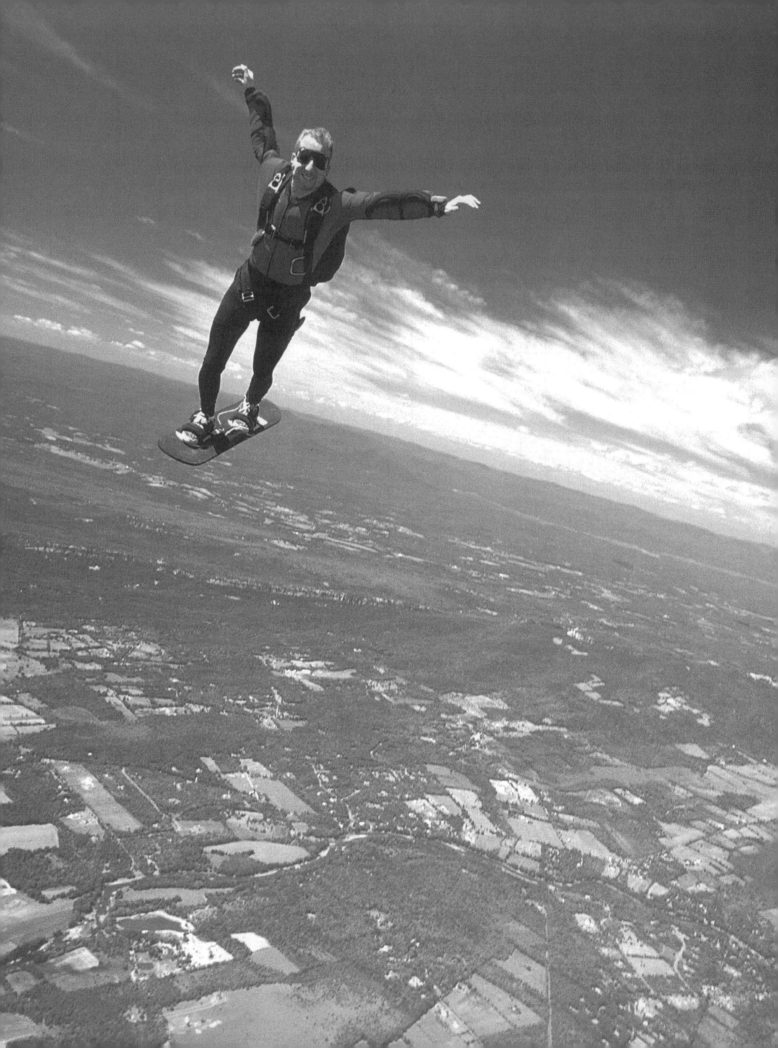

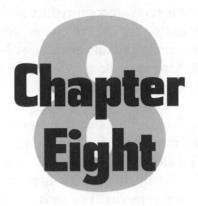

Chapter Eight

Xtreme Spirit—Unleashing The Force Behind True Xcellence

Without question, the X-athlete is the most dedicated athlete in any sport, and his or her pursuit is for the most noble of reasons: the love of the game. The success of making that trick or barreling through that tight wave doesn't come easy. It's earned through hard work, endless hours of practice, and complete conviction.

Thus, the X-athlete who is intent on being the best he or she can be follows the proverbial "road less traveled." And while the pathway to greatness exists, only those who have conviction in their goals will complete the arduous journey. Doing so lies in meeting life's daily challenges—those small, inconspicuous tasks that test you on a regular basis. It's the sum of those tasks that comprise the journey and that make you the best you can be.

Only a handful of athletes are blessed with rare genetic gifts that elicit the perception that they are special. But I prefer to think as special those individuals who dedicate themselves to preparation and attack their loftiest goals. The athletes who continue to push themselves when others slack off or drop out—they are truly the gifted ones, the Renegades. Be assured: There are no posers in the Renegade world! Renegades train hard and ride hard, and in the end, they know they've done their best.

In most athletic coaching circles, the incredible artistry, athleticism, and dedication of the X-athlete is rarely recognized let alone appreciated. But in the world of Renegade Training, the X-athlete is celebrated for his or her incredible talent and unrelenting pursuit of success. Nothing more typifies the Renegade spirit than the Xtreme athlete, who pushes on through the painful lessons of missed jumps and busted tricks.

Throughout this book, I have laid out the blueprint for how to fulfill an athlete's physical potential in training for Xtreme sports. And while the science behind Renegade training can get you there, it's not enough. That's why in this final chapter, I address the X-athlete's spirituality—what lies inside him or her in terms of commitment and integrity. For those qualities will go a long way in determining his or her success. In fact, developing spirituality may be the first step down the pathway to greatness.

What is the source of that commitment? What determines an athlete's resolve or motivation? An attempt to answer these questions would likely stir up the age-old debate of nature versus nurture—that is, whether someone is born with superior athletic ability or has to work for everything. A selected few athletes seem born to play their sport and come equipped with the physical skills and psychological determination to make it happen. Others are raised with a strong work ethic, but that is becoming more and more rare, unfortunately. Thus, training needs to take on the additional purpose of developing the "never say die" attitude that's required to excel. To improve, to be great, you must rise up after a hard fall and force yourself to bust that tough trick.

Throughout my career, I've proven that this relentless attitude can be fostered among athletes, but first, the will and desire must burn within them. Challenge is something that Renegade athletes are accustomed to. Overcoming adversity is part of their daily training. To be successful in their performance arena, whatever that may be, athletes must have intimate knowledge of how to deal with a chaotic environment and how to react instinctively. This is basically a military theory that I adapted for my training programs a long time ago, and the success of my programs has proven its validity. If you train in chaos, it will become your ally.

Will and desire are the foundation of all training, for without the proper psychological development, all physical development will be fruitless. In addition, the following personal attributes are needed to achieve greatness. They are all intertwined and thus mutually dependent and reinforcing. These attributes are genderless, ageless, and without racial or economic barriers:

Integrity: This is the moral fabric of the athlete and thus impacts his or her drive, commitment, and discipline. Qualities such as passion, restraint, and interpersonal skills help form the cornerstone to the spirit of an athlete.

Drive: The insatiable and relentless thirst to succeed is perhaps the most important quality of an athlete. The successful athlete makes progress most efficiently by focusing on and working toward well thought out goals. True drive is unyielding, even in the face of real adversity. One cannot quit until the mission has been accomplished. There is no task that cannot be completed.

Commitment: Renegade Training takes athletes through a comprehensive and brutal workout, in which they are challenged at every turn. Renegade athletes never allow themselves to be vanquished. They face challenges head on and ultimately accomplish their dreams—if they want to. I realize that exercise physiologists will criticize this approach as unsound in academic terms, and they may be accurate in doing so, except for one thing: My athletes learn to defy the challenges set before them, and that learning starts right here! Some might consider this approach as punishment, but that's not my intent. My goal is to make you, and every athlete, better, stronger, and tougher— mentally as well as physically. Pain not only will be denied, but it will become an ally. Losing cannot be considered an option.

Discipline: The disciplined athlete is so committed to achieving his or her goals that he or she considers even those elements beyond training, such as diet and rest. In sum, training must extend to all aspects of one's life that will improve performance. The comprehensive element of discipline is something many athletes do not understand when they commit themselves to training.

Conviction: Conviction may also be called *faith*, but not as it's used in the religious sense. Rather, the appropriate meaning of *faith* for this context is that from the motto of the U.S. Marine Corps, "*Semper fidelis,*" which is Latin for "*Always faithful.*" The athlete who possesses real conviction will have the courage and perseverance to press on during the most difficult times because he or she will know that this it the right course of action.

Making your way along the pathway to greatness is unquestionably a daunting task. But every journey must begin by taking that first step. For the athlete, that first step is to develop his or her mindset—namely, the will and desire to achieve. With that as the foundation for the development of the requisite physical skills, an athlete is surely destined for success.

Every X-athlete, whatever his or her sport, faces enormous challenges everyday—be it to paddle out to a bigger set of waves, to prepare to drop into a higher vert ramp, or to figure out how to charge through a course. Each of these challenges puts the X-athlete to the test, and how he or she responds will determine his or her long-term success.

Understand that no one is going to pick you up and get you going again after you take a spill. It's you and you alone. And that means that what burns inside you is what will push you on.

So, in the very simplest of terms, take control of your destiny. Seize and crush every limitation you see before you. For buried deep with you is greatness!

In faith,
Coach Davies

About the Author

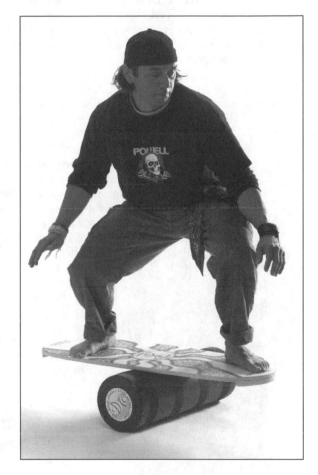

Coach Davies, Coach Davies, renowned as a trainer of some of the world's greatest athletes, is creator of the Renegade school of performance development and author of *Renegade Training for Football*.

His athletes worldwide have accelerated their development beyond what they ever conceived possible and have consistently made themselves known for their ferocious commitment to excellence. Now, after decades of being an active participant in Xtreme sports, Coach Davies brings his brand of training to the board / riding sport genre.

The Renegade instills a warrior mindset in his athletes whether they be on the gridiron or paddling into some serious surf. A take-charge approach to training for the fearless Xtreme athlete is finally available.

To contact the author directly email Coach Davies at:

coachdavies@renegadetraining.com

"Unleash a Shattering, Unstoppable INTENSITY!"

What does it really take to WIN in football?

How can you turn apparent athletic mediocrity into an unstoppable force that can't stop winning?

Why do God-given talents and genetic-freaks so often fail on the field to lesser mortals?

How do you get the victory before you even step on the field?

What fail-safe training method can churn out winners, year-in, year-out, with a staggering consistency?

Enter the secret stealth weapon of modern football success, **Coach Davies**, who has helped high school, college and NFL teams turn lead into gold—and also-rans into number one—with startling frequency. In *Renegade Training for Football*, Coach Davies presents you with his full program for gridiron mastery.

"It's not a game, it's a war!" Coach Davies drills into his athletes. Extreme functional toughness, a bloody-minded brutality of purpose and a nasty-streak one mile wide defines the training mindset.

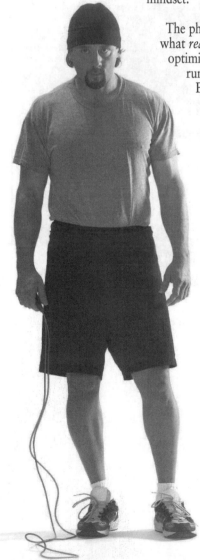

The physical program itself cuts to the core of what *really, really, really* works-in-the-trenches to optimize on-the-field performance. Techniques run the gamut from cutting-edge Eastern European to tried-and-true traditional. It's all here, from rope-skipping, stretching, hurdling, sprint set-up and Olympic lifts to esoteric Russian Kettlebells, abs-work, ladder work, jumping, tumbling and cones. A goldmine of explicit charts and racks of photographs ensure your complete grasp of how to blow past your current athletic level and ratchet up to greatness.

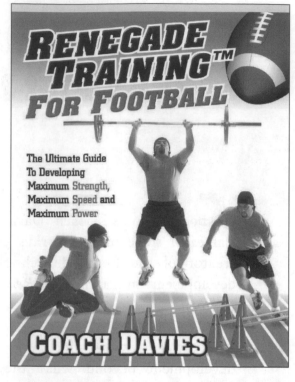

Renegade Training for Football
The Ultimate Guide to Developing Maximum Strength, Maximum Speed and Maximum Power
Book By Coach Davies
Paperback 225 pages 8.5" x 11"
#B21 $34.95

Discover everything YOU need to know for:

- **Range of Motion Development**
- **Agility Training**
- **Linear Speed Development**
- **Strength Development**
- **Work Capacity Development**
- **Spiritual Development**

We'll see YOU in the HALL OF FAME!

About the Author

Coach Davies develops comprehensive training packages for all facets and levels of football, from high school to college to the NFL. Internationally, Coach Davies has been acclaimed for his work with European and South American soccer teams.

His Renegade Training philosophy is controversial but has proved highly successful in application. Coach Davies instills a "warrior mindset" in his athletes. The result: a stand-out toughness capable of excelling in the controlled chaos and extreme stress of modern football. Physically, his athletes have consistently broken through past performance barriers to dramatically enhance their speed, strength and power.

Praise for Coach Davies and Renegade Training

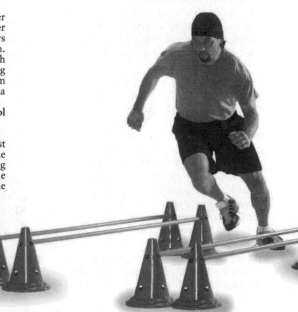

"Our players are in the best shape they've ever been in and they're able to keep up with other teams who a year ago blew past them."

"In my 20 years of coaching, I have been fortunate to have been associated with a lot of top quality coaches. When I think of someone whom I would want to send my kids to for speed and quickness development along with a new approach to overall training methods, the one who comes to mind first and foremost is John Davies. I have personally watched him interact on the field and have had the opportunity to send a lot of my athletes to him and everyone of them have made incredible gains in all aspects. John is unique with his style, he has cutting edge techniques, but what impresses me most is the way he puts things into a simplified and easy to understand methods that can be tailored to athletes at all levels. Undoubtedly you will find John's **Renegade Training for Football** to be both rewarding and refreshing!! Enjoy!!"
—**Steve Mooshagian**, NFL Wide Receivers Coach

"I just wanted to thank you for all of the power-speed programs you have developed for our football program the past two years. We continue to make tremendous progress in the area of speed development and conditioning. The individual programs you have developed by position serves as a motivational tool for our players. Our players have responded well to the position specific training regiments. The blend of 100% sprint work with agility, interval training, resistance sprints, tempo sprints, GPP, SPP, and power-speed drills is truly outstanding. Adding the functional speed-strength work medicine ball drills and sand pit has given us a nice package to work with in developing a faster, powerful athlete. Our staff continues to be amazed at how well our players have progressed through the different levels of the power-speed program. The program emphasizes total athletic development while elevating work capacity and training volumes. The power-speed program demands the best from each player every day during the off-season and pre-season training period."
— **Joey Batson**, SCC, MSS, Director of Strength Speed and Conditioning, **Clemson University**

"Playing football it Canada, you do not receive the same level of coaching that players do in the U.S., and are often left to fend for yourself when it comes to off-season training. Over the years I have tried nearly every 'football specific' workout out there, and found that none of them addressed all of the needs specific to the sport of football. However, Coach Davies' program addresses all of these needs—speed, agility, strength, power and general physical preparation—and puts them into a properly periodized and easy to follow year-round workout program. I have made incredible progress over a short period of time using his workouts, and wish that I had access to his guidance years ago."
—**Scott Vass, Simon Fraser University Clansmen Football**.

"Joining the Renegade Coaching program has made an immediate impact on the young athletes that I work with. As their personal coach I want

the best for them. What better programs to give them than the Renegade Workout? GPP and its proper implementation have made me a believer in any program John Davies creates. I have seen dramatic changes in my athlete's hip flexibility and overall work capacity. Coach Davies training program has launched my athletes' confidence and will to succeed."
—**Dan Fichter**, Wannagetfast, Power Speed Training, Rochester, NY

"John's work is on the cutting edge; it always has been and always will be. He dares to go where few will tread. He attacks athletic performance with a force firmly founded in tradition as well as venturing into what some deem unconventional. In the end, the results speak for themselves. Wins, wins, and more wins. Little more need be said."
— **Mike Ryan**, College and High School football coach, CA

"Coach Davies' concepts on training football players are the best that I have ever encountered! His "renegade style" of training the football athlete is unique to any other form of training. It does not emphasize just one or two aspects of football such as weight training and conditioning; it emphasizes all facets equally, which in turn creates a great player on the gridiron. Explosive strength, agility, quickness, flexibility, special awareness, reaction time, conditioning and most importantly, warrior attitude and mental & physical toughness are all developed fully and given equal attention!"
— **Derek Alford**, Offensive Coordinator/Quarterbacks, **Garland High School**, TX.

"John Davies is the new wizard of innovation in sport-specific training. If you don't read this book, then winning must not be very important to you."
—**Arik Orosz**, Trainer, Minneapolis, MN

"Our players are in the best shape they've ever been in and they're able to keep up with other teams who a year ago blew past them. The boys have a love/hate relationship with the program. They believe in it and are willing to go through it, but they also admit that it's the toughest thing they've ever done. They know it will make them better athletes as well as people. If you're gonna be a bear, be a grizzly."
— **Jabo Burgess**, Coach, **Easley High School** Easley, SC

"Working with Coach Davies was been the most intense experience in both the training and the results that I have had since starting training twenty years ago. I have become a true "Renegade." I now prefer to train alone after the gym closes by myself, leaving my training partners wondering what has caused my new found level of speed, strength and endurance."
— **Jay Cox**, Deputy Sheriff, Bishopville, MD

"I have learned more in seven months from Coach Davies about the practical application of exercises and hard work in the real world than I did from the other "experts" in 17 years lifting, a Master's degree in Exercise Physiology, countless journals and magazines."
— **Kevin Herring**, Birmingham, AL

"Most strength coaches and football athletes have confused football conditioning with weight lifting. The ability to bench press the weight room has little positive transfer to the playing arena. Fortunately, John Davies' new book on football conditioning will provide the proper roadmap for the aspiring football athlete and his strength coach. The depth of Coach Davies' experience with the football athlete combined with his in-depth knowledge is rarely found in today's contemporary coach. I have found him to be an invaluable resource. His workouts are not only a tremendous challenge that produces results, but they provide a refreshing perspective on this modern gizmo, no pain and no gain mentality. I would not hesitate to recommend this book to any athlete or conditioning consultant."
— **Michael Rutherford**, M.S. Exercise Physiology.

"Coach Davies is the real deal. After three months of training under his guidance, I was able to reach levels of strength and speed that I never thought would've been possible. I'm much more confident in my skills as an athlete and can't wait to be able to apply them to the football field in a few months."
—**M.J. Mafaro**, Staten Island, NY.

ANNOUNCING:
"The World's *Single Most Effective Tool* for Massive Gains in Strength, Speed and Athletic Endurance"

Discover why Russian Kettlebells are storming into "favored status" with US military, SWAT, NFL, MLB, powerlifters, weightlifters, martial artists—and elite athletes everywhere.

- Get thick, cable-like, hellaciously hard muscle
- Get frightening, whip-like speed
- Get stallion-like staying-power in any sport
- Get a, well, <u>god-like</u> physique
- Get the most brutal workout of your life, without having to leave your own living room
- Get way more energy in way less time
- Get a jack-rabbit's jumping power—and a jack-hammer's strength
- Get it all—and then more, with Russian KB's

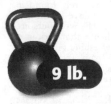 **9 lb.**   **18 lb.** 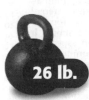 **26 lb.**   **35 lb.**   **53 lb.**   **70 lb.** 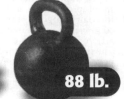 **88 lb.**

KETTLEBELLS DESIGNED FOR WOMEN

Each authentic Russian Kettlebell is manufactured exclusively by Dragon Door Publications in traditional weight sizes. The kettlebells are made out of solid cast iron and are coated in the highest quality scratch and rust resistant cathodic epoxy gloss. These kettlebells are designed to last a lifetime—and beyond.

Special warning: the *Russian Kettlebell* is an *Xtreme Edge Fitness* Tool for serious workout fiends. It is not a Barbie toy! Treat your kettlebell lifting with the utmost care, precision and respect. Watch Pavel's kettlebell video many, many times for perfect form and correct execution. If possible, sign up for one of Pavel's upcoming Kettlebell Training Bootcamp/ Certification programs. Lift at your own discretion! We are not responsible for you boinking yourself on the head, dropping it on your feet or any other politically-incorrect action. Stick to the Party line, Comrade!

CLASSIC KETTLEBELLS

RUSSIAN KETTLEBELLS

SIZES DESIGNED FOR WOMEN

#P10D	4kg (approx. 9 lb)	$89.95 S/H: $10.00
#P10E	8kg (approx. 18 lb)	$99.95 S/H: $14.00

Until further notice, these new kettlebells are not available as a set.

CLASSIC KETTLEBELLS

#P10G	12kg (approx. 26lb)	$82.95 S/H: $20.00
#P10A	16kg (approx. 35lb)	$89.95 S/H: $24.00
#P10B	24kg (approx. 53lb)	$109.95 S/H: $32.00
#P10C	32kg (approx. 70lb)	$139.95 S/H: $39.00

NEW! 40kg SIZE—HEAVY METAL!

#P10F 40kg (approx. 88lb) $179.95 S/H: $52.00

SAVE! ORDER A SET OF CLASSIC KETTLEBELLS AND SAVE $17.00!

#SP10 Set, one of A, B & C—16, 24 & 32kg. (Save $17.00) $322.85 S/H: $95.00

The Russian Kettlebells are only available to customers resident in the U.S. mainland. Normal shipping charges do not apply. No rush orders on kettlebells.

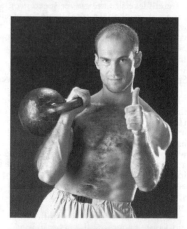

1•800•899•5111
24 HOURS A DAY
FAX YOUR ORDER
(866) 280-7619

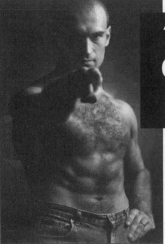
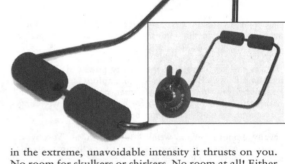
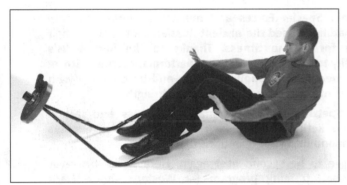
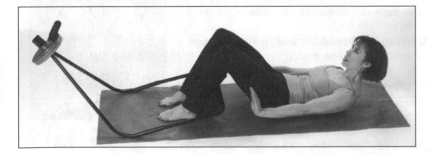

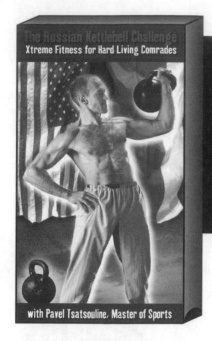

The Russian Kettlebell Challenge

Xtreme Fitness for Hard Living Comrades

with Pavel Tsatsouline, Master of Sports

Video Item # V103 • $39.95 or DVD Item # DV001 • $39.95
Running Time: 32 minutes

An ancient Russian exercise device, the kettlebell has long been a favorite in that country for those seeking a special edge in strength and endurance.

It was the key in forging the mighty power of dinosaurs like Ivan "the Champion of Champions", Poddubny. Poddubny, one of the strongest men of his time, trained with kettlebells in preparation for his undefeated wrestling career and six world champion belts.

Many famous Soviet weightlifters, such as Vorobyev, Vlasov, Alexeyev, and Stogov, started their Olympic careers with old-fashioned kettlebells.

Kettlebells come in "poods". A pood is an old Russian measure of weight, which equals 16kg, or 36 pounds. There are one, one and a half, and two pood K-bells, 16, 24, and 32kg respectively.

To earn his national ranking, Pavel Tsatsouline had to power snatch a 32kg kettlebell forty times with one arm, and forty with the other back to back and power clean and jerk two such bells forty-five times.

Soviet science discovered that repetition kettlebell lifting is one of the best tools for all around physical development. (Voropayev, 1983) observed two groups of college students over a period of a few years. A standard battery of the armed forces PT tests was used: pullups, a standing broad jump, a 100m sprint, and a 1k run. The control groupfollowed the typical university physical training program which was military oriented and emphasized the above exercises. The experimental group just lifted kettlebells. In spite of the lack of practice on the tested drills, the KB group showed better scores in every one of them.

The Red Army, too pragmatic to waste their troopers, time on pushups and situps, quickly caught on. Every Russian military unit's gym was equipped with K-bells. Spetznaz, Soviet Special Operations, personnel owe much of their wiry strength, explosive agility, and never quitting stamina to kettlebells. High rep C&Js and snatches with K-bells kick the fighting man,s system into warp drive.

In addition to their many mentioned benefits, the official kettlebell lifts also develop the ability to absorb ballistic shocks. If you want to develop your ability to take impact try the official K-bell lifts. The repetitive ballistic shock builds extremely strong tendons and ligaments.

The ballistic blasts of kettlebell lifting become an excellent conditioning tool for athletes from rough sports like kick boxing, wrestling, and football. And the extreme metabolic cost of high rep KB workouts will put your unwanted fat on a fire sale.

If you are looking for a supreme edge in your chosen sport—seek no more!

Both the Soviet Special Forces and numerous world-champion Soviet Olympic athletes used the ancient Russian Kettlebell as their secret weapon for xtreme fitness. Thanks to the kettlebells's astonishing ability to turbocharge physical performance, these Soviet supermen creamed their opponents time-and-time-again, with inhuman displays of raw power and explosive strength.

Now, former Spetznaz trainer, international fitness author and nationally ranked kettlebell lifter, Pavel Tsatsouline, delivers this secret Soviet weapon into your own hands.

You **NEVER have to be second best again!** Here is the first-ever complete kettlebell training program—for Western shock-attack athletes who refuse to be denied—and who'd rather be dead than number two.

- Get really, really nasty—with a commando's wiry strength, the explosive agility of a tiger and the stamina of a world-class ironman.

- Own the single best conditioning tool for killer sports like kickboxing, wrestling, and football.

- Watch in amazement as high-rep kettlebells let you hack the fat off your meat—without the dishonor of aerobics and dieting

- Kick your fighting system into warp speed—with high-rep snatches and clean-and-jerks

- Develop steel tendons and ligaments—and a whiplash power to match

- Effortlessly absorb ballistic shocks—and laugh as you shrug off the hardest hits your opponent can muster

- Go ape on your enemies—with gorilla shoulders and tree-swinging traps

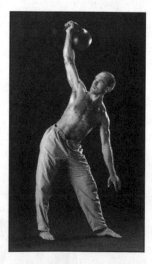

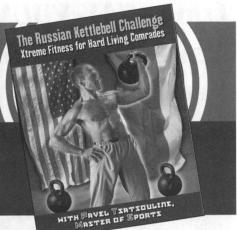
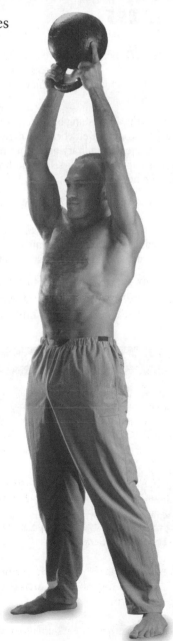
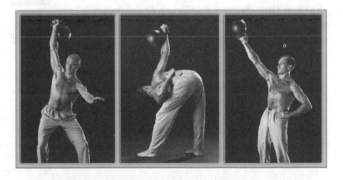

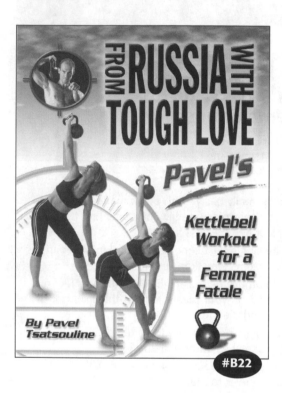

"Download this tape into your eager cells and watch in stunned disbelief as your body reconstitutes itself, almost overnight"

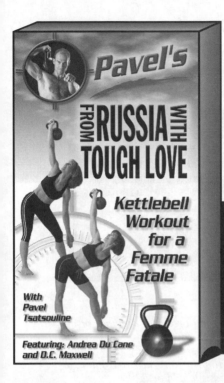

With Pavel Tsatsouline

Featuring: Andrea Du Cane and D.C. Maxwell

From Russia with Tough Love

Pavel's Kettlebell Workout
for a Femme Fatale
With Pavel Tsatsouline
Running Time: 1hr 12 minutes
Video #V110 $29.95
DVD #DV002 $29.95

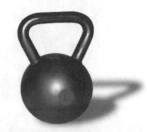

The Sure-Fire Secret to Looking Younger, Leaner and Stronger <u>AND</u> Having More Energy to Get a Whole Lot More Done in the Day

What you'll discover when "Tough" explodes on your monitor:

- The *Snatch*—to eliminate cellulite, firm your butt, and give you the cardio-workout of a lifetime
- The *Swing*— to fry your fat and slenderize hips 'n thighs
- The *Power Breathing Crunch*—to shrink your waist
- The *Deck Squat*—for strength and super-flexiblity
- An incredible exercise to tone your arms and shoulders
- The *Clean-and-Press*—for a magnificent upper body
- The *Overhead Squat*—for explosive leg strength
- The queen of situps—for a flat, flat stomach
- Combination exercises that wallop you with an unbelievable muscular and cardio workout

Spanking graphics, a kick-ass opening, smooth-as-silk camera work, Pavel at his absolute dynamic best, two awesome femme fatales, and a slew of fantastic KB exercises, many of which were not included on the original Russian Kettlebell Challenge video.

At one hour and twenty minutes of rock-solid, cutting-edge information, this video is value-beyond-belief. I challenge any woman worth her salt not to be able to completely transform herself physically with this one tape.

"In six weeks of kettlebell work, I lost an inch off my waist and dropped my heart rate 6 beats per minute, while staying the same weight. I was already working out when I started using kettlebells, so I'm not a novice. There are few ways to lose fat, gain muscle, and improve your cardio fitness all at the same time; I've never seen a better one than this."
—*Steven Justus, Westminster, CO*

"Kettlebells are without a doubt the most effective strength/endurance conditioning tool out there. I wish I had known about them 15 years ago!"
—*Santiago, Orlando, FL*

"I have practiced Kettlebell training for a year and a half. I now have an anatomy chart back and have gotten MUCH stronger."
—*Samantha Mendelson, Coral Gables, FL*

"I know now that I will never walk into a gym again - who would? It is absolutely amazing how much individual accomplishment can be attained using a kettlebell. Simply fantastic. I would recommend it to anyone at any fitness level, in any sport.
—*William Hevener, North Cape May, NJ*

"It is the most effective training tool I have ever used. I have increased both my speed and endurance, with extra power to boot. It wasn't even a priority, but I lost some bodyfat, which was nice. However, increased athletic performance was my main goal, and this is where the program really shines."
—*Tyler Hass, Walla Walla, WA*

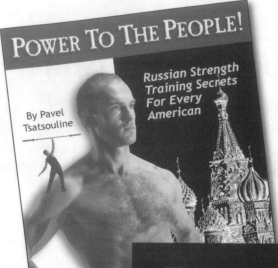

"*Power to the People! is absolute dynamite. If there was only one book I could recommend to help you reach your ultimate physical potential, this would be it.*"

—Jim Wright, Ph.D., Science Editor, Flex Magazine, Weider Group

POWER TO THE PEOPLE!

RUSSIAN STRENGTH TRAINING SECRETS FOR EVERY AMERICAN

By Pavel Tsatsouline

8½" x 11" 124 pages, over 100 photographs and illustrations—$34.95 #B10

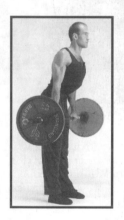

How would you like to own a world class body—<u>whatever your present condition</u>— by doing only two exercises, for twenty minutes a day?" A body so lean, ripped and powerful looking, you won't believe your own reflection when you catch yourself in the mirror.

And what if you could do it without a single supplement, without having to waste your time at a gym and with only a 150 bucks of simple equipment?

And how about not only being stronger than you've ever been in your life, but having higher energy and better performance in whatever you do?

How would you like to have an instant download of the world's <u>absolutely most effective strength secrets?</u> To possess exactly the same knowledge that created world-champion athletes—and the strongest bodies of their generation?"

Pavel Tsatsouline's *Power to the People!— Russian Strength Training Secrets for Every American* delivers all of this and more.

As Senior Science Editor for Joe Weider's *Flex* magazine, Jim Wright is recognized as one of the world's premier authorities on strength training. Here's more of what he had to say:

"*Whether you're young or old, a beginner or an elite athlete, training in your room or in the most high tech facility, if there was only one book I could recommend to help you reach your ultimate physical potential, this would be it.*

Simple, concise and truly reader friendly, this amazing book contains it all—everything you need to know—what exercises (only two!), how to do them (unique detailed information you'll find nowhere else), and why.

Follow its advice and, believe it or not, you'll be stronger and more injury-resistant immediately. I guarantee it. I only wish I'd had a book like this when I first began training.

Follow this program for three months and you'll not only be amazed but hooked. It is the ultimate program for "Everyman" AND Woman! I thought I knew a lot with a Ph.D. and 40 years of training experience...but I learned a lot and it's improved my training significantly."

And how about this from World Masters Powerlifting champion and Parrillo Performance Press editor, Marty Gallagher:

"*Pavel Tsatsouline has burst onto the American health and fitness scene like a Russian cyclone. He razes the sacred temples of fitness complacency and smugness with his revolutionary concepts and ideas. If you want a new and innovative approach to the age old dilemma of physical transformation, you've struck the mother-lode.*"

Here's just some of what you'll discover, when you possess your own copy of Pavel Tsatsouline's *Power to the People!*:

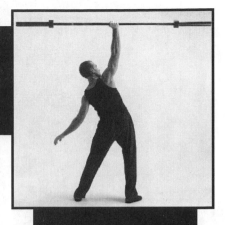

- How to get super strong without training to muscle failure or exhaustion
- How to hack into your 'muscle software' and magnify your power and muscle definition
- How to get super strong <u>without putting on an ounce of weight</u>
- Or how to build massive muscles with a classified Soviet Special Forces workout
- Why high rep training to the 'burn' is like a form of rigor mortis—and what it really takes to develop spectacular muscle tone
- How to mold your whole body into an off-planet rock with only two exercises
- How to increase your bench press by ten pounds overnight
- How to get a tremendous workout on the road without any equipment
- How to design a world class body in your basement—with $150 worth of basic weights and in twenty minutes a day
- How futuristic techniques can squeeze more horsepower out of your body-engine
- How to maximize muscular tension for traffic-stopping muscular definition
- How to minimize fatigue and get the most out of your strength training
- How to ensure high energy after your workout
- How to get stronger and harder without getting bigger
- Why it's safer to use free weights than machines
- How to achieve massive muscles <u>and</u> awesome strength—if that's what you want
- What, how and when to eat for maximum gains
- How to master the magic of effective exercise variation
- The ultimate formula for strength
- How to gain beyond your wildest dreams—with less chance of injury
- A high intensity, immediate gratification technique for massive strength gains
- The eight most effective breathing habits for lifting weights
- The secret that separates elite athletes from 'also-rans'

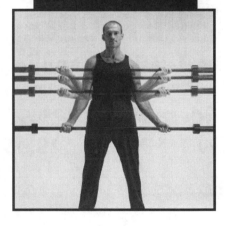

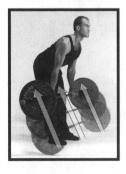

Russians have always made do with simple solutions without compromising the results. NASA aerospace types say that while America sends men to the moon in a Cadillac, Russia manages to launch them into space in a tin can. Enter the tin can approach to designing a world class body—in your basement with $150 worth of equipment. After all, US gyms are stuffed with hi-tech gear, yet it is the Russians with their

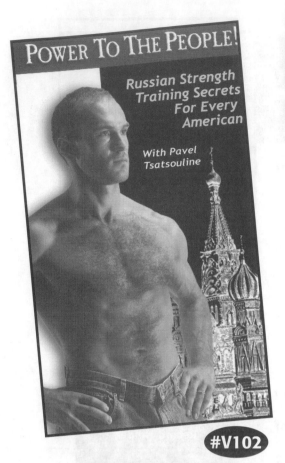

POWER TO THE PEOPLE!

Russian Strength
Training Secrets
For Every
American

With Pavel
Tsatsouline

#V102

POWER TO
THE PEOPLE

By Pavel Tsatsouline
Running time: 47 min

Video #V102 $29.95
DVD #DV004 $29.95

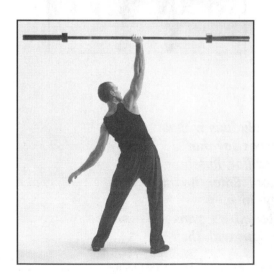

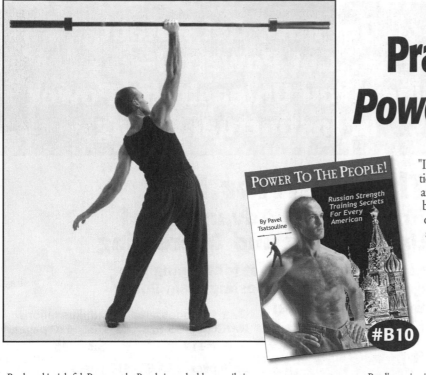

Praise for Pavel's *Power to the People!*

"In **Power to the People!** Pavel Tsatsouline reveals an authentically Russian approach to physical fitness. He shows how anyone, by learning how to contract their muscles harder, can build up to incredible levels of strength without gaining an ounce of weight. He shows how to exercise with a super-strict form and lift more weight than can be accomplished by swing or cheat. Now it's possible to train the human body to world-class fitness standards at home, working out for twenty minutes a day, and with only $150.00 worth of basic weights. **Power to the People!** is a highly recommended addition to any personal or professional physical fitness reference bookshelf."—**Midwest Book Review**, Oregon, WI

Brash and insightful, Power to the People is a valuable compilation of how-to strength training information. Pavel Tsatsouline offers a fresh and provocative perspective on resistance training, and charts a path to self-improvement that is both practical and elegantly simple. If building strength is your top priority, then *Power to the People* belongs at the top of your reading list. —**Rob Faigin, author of Natural Hormonal Enhancement**

"I learned a lot from Pavel's books and plan to use many of his ideas in my own workouts. *Power to the People!* is an eye-opener. It will give you new—and valuable—perspectives on strength training. You will find plenty of ideas here to make your training more productive."—**Clarence Bass, author of Ripped 1, 2 &3.**

"A good book for the athlete looking for a routine that will increase strength without building muscle mass. Good source of variation for anyone who's tired of doing standard exercises."—**Jonathan Lawson, IronMan Magazine**

"I have been a training athlete for over 30 years. I played NCAA basketball in college, kick boxed as a pro for two years, made it to the NFL as a free agent in 1982, powerlifted through my 20's and do Olympic lifting now at 42. I have also coached swimming and strength athletes for over 20 years.I have never read a book more useful than **Power to the People!** I have seen my strength explode like I was in my 20's again—and my joints are no longer hurting."—**Carter Stamm, New Orleans, LA**

"I have been following a regimen I got from *Power to the People!* for about seven weeks now. I have lost about 17lbs and have lost three inches in my waist. My deadlift has gone from a meager 180lbs to 255 lbs in that short time as well."—**Lawrence J. Kochert**

"Like *Beyond Stretching* and *Beyond Crunches*, his other books, this is great. I think that it is the best book on effective strength training that I have ever read. This is not a book just about theory and principles. But Tsatsouline provides a detailed and complete outline of an exact program to do and how to customize it for yourself. It is very different from anything you have probably every read about strength training. The things he teaches in the book though won't just get you strong, if you want more than that, but can make you look really good—lean, ripped, and/or real big muscled if you want it. It's a very good book; the best available English-language print matter on the topic of strength training."—**Dan Paltzik**

"The great thing about the book *"Power to the People!"* is that it tells the readers what not to do when training for strength and why not. As you read the book, you will keep saying to yourself: "so that's why I'm not getting stronger!" Pavel points out all the things that are wrong with conventional weight training (and there is lots of it) and shows the readers what they need to do to get stronger, but not necessarily bigger."— **Sang Kim, Rome, GA**

"Using Pavel Tsatsouline's weight training methods from his book *Power to the People* gives you the feeling that you can take on the world after only a 20-30 minute workout! Tsatsouline's book is written with such cleverness, clarity, and detail that I couldn't put it down. I am thoroughly enthusiastic about weight training where my past indoor training consisted only of Yoga postures. I would recommend this book to anyone interested in enhancing their performance on the job, in weight training, and in other athletic pursuits.

Pavel's genius is that he can take a complex subject like weight training and design a program that is enjoyable, efficient and gets fast results. He has done the same thing for abdominal development and stretching."—**Cliff D.V., Honolulu, Hawaii**

"I have experienced Pavel Tsatsouline's methods up close and in person, and his scientific approach lays waste to the muscleheaded garbage that we've been conditioned to follow. Pavel will show you how to achieve a full-body workout with just two core exercises and $150 worth of barbell equipment. You won't get injured and you won't get stiff. You'll just get what you were looking for in the first place - a program that works and one that you'll stick with." — **David M Gaynes, Bellevue, WA**

"It isn't growth hormone... it's Pavel! This is THE definitive text on the art and science of strength training... and that's what it's all about, power! Page after page of the world's most useful and productive strength-training practices are explained in this book. A lot of experienced lifters, who think that they know how to train, will be humbled when they find out how much better Pavel's system is than anything the western iron-game community has ever done. I have surpassed all my previous bests...and I no longer need or use lifting belts. I learned how to up-regulate tension through his "feed-forward" technique, how to immediately add AT LEAST ten pounds to every lift via "hyperirradiation", and to do it in my best form ever, and how to gain on every lift WEEKLY through the Russian system of periodization without any plateaus! Seriously, I gain every week! You only need TWO exercises! Pavel explains which ones, how to do them and how often. Also, you'll learn how to train to SUCCESS, not to "failure", how to immediately turn any lift into a "hyper lift", teach your nervous system how not to ever "miss" a lift, and simultaneously make your body far less injury-prone! Pavel illustrates the two types of muscle growth and which one you REALLY need, and the all-important power breathing. Pavel's training is the most valuable resource made available for strength athletes since the barbell. The breathing techniques alone are worth the asking price. This book is my personal favorite out of all his works, and in my opinion, they should be owned as a set. This book is superior to all the muscle mags and books that dwell on a content of unessential details of today's "fitness culture" and yet never fully explain the context of training for strength. Pavel cuts right to the heart of the "muscle mystery", by explaining the all-important context of the Russian system: quick, efficient, permanent strength gains, without spending a small fortune on "me-too" bodybuilding supplements and without unnecessary, time consuming overtraining. Now I only hope he writes a book on full-contact training..."—**Sean Williams, Long Beach, NY**

"This is a real source of no-b.s. information on how to build strength without adding bulk. I learned some new things which one can't find in books like *'Beyond Brawn'* or *'Dinosaur Training'*. Perhaps an advanced powerlifter, who reads Milo, already knows all that stuff, but I would definitely recommend this book to everyone from beginners to intermediates who are interested in increasing their strength." —**Nikolai Pastouchenko, Tallahassee, Florid**

"Forget all of the fancy rhetoric. If you are serious about improving your strength and your health buy this book and pay attention to what's provided. I started in January 2000 doing deadlifts with 200 lbs. Three months later I was at 365 lbs. Pavel knows what he is talking about and knows how to explain it simply. That's it."—**Alan, Indiana**

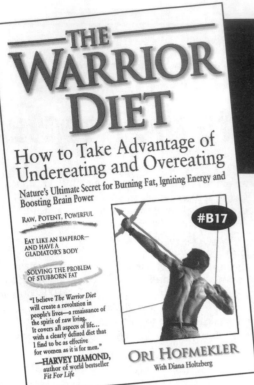

Eat like an emperor—and have a gladiator's body

Are you still confused about what, how and when to eat? Despite the diet books you have read and the programs you have tried, do you still find yourself lacking in energy, carrying excess body fat, and feeling physically run-down? Sexually, do you feel a shadow of your former self?

The problem, according to **Ori Hofmekler,** is that we have lost touch with the natural wisdom of our instinctual drives. We have become the slaves of our own creature comforts—scavenger/victims rather than predator/victors. When to comes to informed-choice, we lack any real sense of personal freedom. The result: ill-advised eating and lifestyle habits that leave us vulnerable to all manner of disease—not to mention obesity and sub-par performance.

The Warrior Diet presents a brilliant and far-reaching solution to our nutritional woes, based on a return to the primal power of our natural instincts.

The first step is to break the chains of our current eating habits. Drawing on a combination of ancient history and modern science, *The Warrior Diet* proves that humans are at their energetic, physical, mental and passionate best when they "undereat" during the day and "overeat" at night. Once you master this essential eating cycle, a new life of explosive vigor and vitality will be yours for the taking.

Unlike so many dietary gurus, Ori Hofmekler has personally followed his diet for over twenty-five years and is a perfect model of *the Warrior Diet's* success—the man is a human dynamo.

Not just a diet, but a whole way of life, *the Warrior Diet* encourages us to seize back the pleasures of being alive—from the most refined to the wild and raw. *The Warrior Diet* is practical, tested, and based in commonsense. Expect results!

The Warrior Diet covers all the bases. As an added bonus, discover delicious Warrior Recipes, a special Warrior Workout, and a line of Warrior Supplements—designed to give you every advantage in the transformation of your life from average to exceptional.

> "I believe *The Warrior Diet* will create a revolution in people's lives— a renaissance of the spirit of raw living. It covers all aspects of life…with a clearly defined diet that I find to be as effective for women as it is for men."
> —**Harvey Diamond,** author of world bestseller *Fit For Life*

> "Rare in books about foods, there is wisdom in the pages of *The Warrior Diet* …Ori knows the techniques, but he shows you a possibility—a platform for living your life as well…*The Warrior Diet* is a book that talks to all of you— the whole person hidden inside."
> —**Udo Erasmus,** author of *Fats That Heal, Fats That Kill*

About Ori Hofmekler

Ori Hofmekler is a modern Renaissance man whose life has been driven by two passions: art and sports. Hofmekler's formative experience as a young man with the Israeli Special Forces, prompted a lifetime's interest in diets and fitness regimes that would optimize his physical and mental performance.

After the army, Ori attended the Bezalel Academy of Art and the Hebrew University, where he studied art and philosophy and received a degree in Human Sciences.

A world-renowned painter, best known for his controversial political satire, Ori's work has been featured in magazines worldwide, including *Time, Newsweek, Rolling Stone, People, The New Republic* as well as *Penthouse* where he was a monthly columnist for 17 years and Health Editor from 1998–2000. Ori has published two books of political art, *Hofmekler's People,* and *Hofmekler's Gallery.*

As founder, Editor-In-Chief, and Publisher of *Mind & Muscle Power,* a national men's health and fitness magazine, Ori introduced his Warrior Diet to the public in a monthly column—to immediate acclaim from readers and professionals in the health industry alike.

ORDERING INFORMATION

Customer Service Questions? Please call us between 9:00am–11:00pm EST Monday to Friday at 1-800-899-5111. Local and foreign customers call 513-346-4160 for orders and customer service

100% One-Year Risk-Free Guarantee. If you are not completely satisfied with any product–for any reason, no matter how long after you received it–we'll be happy to give you a prompt exchange, credit, or refund, as you wish. Simply return your purchase to us, and please let us know why you were dissatisfied–it will help us to provide better products and services in the future. *Shipping and handling fees are non-refundable.*

Telephone Orders For faster service you may place your orders by calling Toll Free 24 hours a day, 7 days a week, 365 days per year. When you call, please have your credit card ready.

1·800·899·5111
24 HOURS A DAY
FAX YOUR ORDER (866) 280-7619

Complete and mail with full payment to: Dragon Door Publications, P.O. Box 1097, West Chester, OH 45071

Please print clearly

Sold To: **A**

Name_____

Street _____

City _____

State _____ Zip _____

Day phone*_____
* Important for clarifying questions on orders

Please print clearly

SHIP TO: *(Street address for delivery)*   **B**

Name_____

Street _____

City _____

State _____ Zip _____

Email _____

ITEM #	QTY.	ITEM DESCRIPTION	ITEM PRICE	A OR B	TOTAL

HANDLING AND SHIPPING CHARGES • NO COD'S
Total Amount of Order Add:

$00.00 to $24.99 add $5.00	$100.00 to $129.99 add $12.00
$25.00 to $39.99 add $6.00	$130.00 to $169.99 add $14.00
$40.00 to $59.99 add $7.00	$170.00 to $199.99 add $16.00
$60.00 to $99.99 add $10.00	$200.00 to $299.99 add $18.00
	$300.00 and up add $20.00

Canada & Mexico add $8.00. All other countries triple U.S. charges.

Total of Goods	
Shipping Charges	
Rush Charges	
Kettlebell Shipping Charges	
OH residents add 6% sales tax	
MN residents add 6.5% sales tax	
TOTAL ENCLOSED	

METHOD OF PAYMENT ❏ CHECK ❏ M.O. ❏ MASTERCARD ❏ VISA ❏ DISCOVER ❏ AMEX

Account No. *(Please indicate all the numbers on your credit card)*   EXPIRATION DATE

❏❏❏❏ ❏❏❏❏ ❏❏❏❏ ❏❏❏❏   ❏❏/❏❏

Day Phone (   ) _____

SIGNATURE _____ DATE _____

NOTE: We ship best method available for your delivery address. Foreign orders are sent by air. Credit card or International M.O. only. For rush processing of your order, add an additional $10.00 per address. Available on money order & charge card orders only.

Errors and omissions excepted. Prices subject to change without notice.

Warning to foreign customers:
The Customs in your country may or may not tax or otherwise charge you an additional fee for goods you receive. Dragon Door Publications is charging you only for U.S. handling and international shipping. Dragon Door Publications is in no way responsible for any additional fees levied by Customs, the carrier or any other entity.

Warning!
This may be the last issue of the catalog you receive.

If we rented your name, or you haven't ordered in the last two years you may not hear from us again. If you wish to stay informed about products and services that can make a difference to your health and well-being, please indicate below.

Name_____

Address_____

City_____ State_____ Zip_____

Phone_____

Do You Have A Friend Who'd Like To Receive This Catalog?

We would be happy to send your friend a free copy. Make sure to print and complete in full:

Name_____

Address_____

City_____ State_____ Zip_____

DDP 06/03

Attack-Dog Toughness, Cat-Like Balance, Razor-Sharp Reactions, Explosive Jump-Ability—Get It All When You Train Xtreme Sports, The Renegade Style

Watcha want? Are you for real? Are you a doer? Can you excel? Do you have what it takes? Can you hack it?

Ready to put muscle in your madness? Fire in your veins? Iron in your claws?

If not, then drop this book and get out of the way! Now!

But if you're seriously afflicted with the burning desire to succeed at all costs, to blow the roof off your past achievements and live like it was your last minute on earth, then grab this thing and make it yours from the inside out.

Welcome, friend, to the style of Renegade. Adopt the code, make it yours and explode to ridiculous new levels of spectacular performance—no question.

Welcome, friend, to the first-ever, complete training program for superlative results in the xtreme sport of your choice.

"You Ain't In The Game If You Ain't Doing It Renegade"

- Perform tricks and feats that'd rock the brain of a digital wiz
- Soar like an eagle—with impossibly high jumps and absurdly extended hang times
- Take Nature's toughest pounding— and bounce away laughing
- Astound competitors with your blazing speed— appall them with your brutal endurance
- Rip the most wicked waves with breathless ease and grace
- Unleash the beast within—on an unsuspecting world
- Cry victory—it's yours for the seizing

Dragon Door Publications, Inc.

www.dragondoor.com

**Visit the Dragon Door website today.
Sign up as a subscriber and
receive free downloads of articles,
news of new products and much more.**

0-938045-51-2 $34.95

ISBN 0-938045-51-2

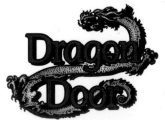

9 780938 045519

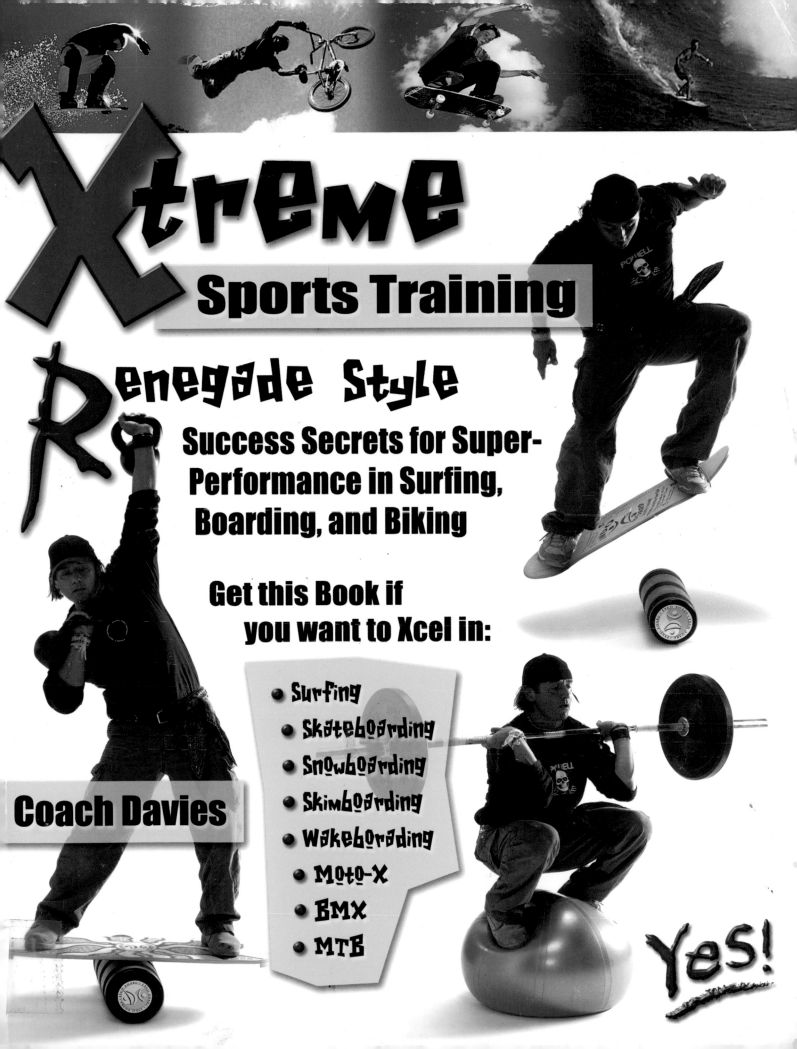